100 Questions & Answers About Autism:
Expert Advice from a Physician/Parent Caregiver

Campion Quinn, MD, MHA
Internist and Medical Consultant
Rockville Centre, NY

JONES AND BARTLETT PUBLISHERS
Sudbury, Massachusetts
BOSTON   TORONTO   LONDON   SINGAPORE

World Headquarters
Jones and Bartlett
Publishers
40 Tall Pine Drive
Sudbury, MA 01776
info@jbpub.com
www.jbpub.com

Jones and Bartlett
Publishers Canada
2406 Nikanna Road
Mississauga, ON
L5C 2W6
CANADA

Jones and Bartlett
Publishers International
Barb House, Barb Mews
London W6 7PA
UK

Jones and Bartlett's books and products are available through most bookstores and online booksellers. To contact Jones and Bartlett Publishers directly, call 800-832-0034, fax 978-443-8000, or visit our website www.jbpub.com.

Substantial discounts on bulk quantities of Jones and Bartlett's publications are available to corporations, professional associations, and other qualified organizations. For details and specific discount information, contact the special sales department at Jones and Bartlett via the above contact information or send an email to specialsales@jbpub.com.

Library of Congress Cataloging-in-Publication Data
Quinn, Campion E.
  100 questions and answers about autism : expert advice from a physician/
parent caregiver / Campion E. Quinn.
    p. cm.
Includes bibliographical references and index.
  ISBN 0-7637-3894-8 (alk. paper)
  1. Autism in children—Miscellanea. 2. Parents of autistic children—Miscellanea.
I. Title. II. Title: One hundred questions and answers about autism.
  RJ506.A9Q85 2006
  618.92'85882—dc22

                                                    2005022351
                                                    6048

Production Credits
Executive Publisher: Christopher Davis
Associate Editor: Kathy Richardson
Production Editor: Karen Ferreira
Associate Marketing Manager: Laura Kavigian
Cover Design: Philip Regan

Manufacturing Buyer: Therese Connell
Composition: Modern Graphics
Printing and Binding: Malloy Lithographing
Cover Printer: Malloy Lithographing

The authors, editor, and publisher have made every effort to provide accurate information. However, they are not responsible for errors, omissions, or for any outcomes related to the use of the contents of this book and take no responsibility for the use of the products described. Treatments and side effects described in this book may not be applicable to all patients; likewise, some patients may require a dose or experience a side effect that is not described herein. The reader should confer with his or her own physician regarding specific treatments and side effects. Drugs and medical devices are discussed that may have limited availability controlled by the Food and Drug Administration (FDA) for use only in a research study or clinical trial. The drug information presented has been derived from reference sources, recently published data, and pharmaceutical research data. Research, clinical practice, and government regulations often change the accepted standard in this field. When consideration is being given to use of any drug in the clinical setting, the health care provider or reader is responsible for determining FDA status of the drug, reading the package insert, reviewing prescribing information for the most up-to-date recommendations on dose, precautions, and contraindications, and determining the appropriate usage for the product. This is especially important in the case of drugs that are new or seldom used.

Printed in the United States of America
09 08 07 06 05   10 9 8 7 6 5 4 3 2 1

This book is dedicated to my son,
Campion.

This book was improved immeasurably by the honest comments and practical insights provided by William and Rebecca Devlin. Their many remarks are found within the text in italics.

Nancy DiPilli and Anthony and Maura Calio also reviewed the text and offered helpful suggestions.

All of them know the joys and challenges of parenting an autistic child. They have my deepest thanks and undying respect.

Autism is not a death sentence.

*Autism is not
a death
sentence.*

Six years ago, after several months of visiting several medical specialists and undergoing blood tests, CTs, EEGs, and audiograms, a neurologist finally diagnosed my only son, Campion, with autism.

At first I didn't believe the doctor who made the diagnosis. Clearly, I thought, this doctor was incompetent. A more skillful doctor could find an easy answer to my son's disturbing symptoms. I looked for that enlightened doctor for several more months. Many doctors examined him. However, the diagnosis remained the same: autism.

I'm a physician; my wife is a nurse. We have two other "typical" children—daughters, who are bright and vivacious. We noticed that although our son achieved most of his developmental milestones, he was unlike his sisters. He didn't speak much, didn't make eye contact with us, and didn't like to be held or cuddled. Autism was the diagnosis we feared; the one that my wife and I would not speak aloud, even to each other. However, the diagnosis was confirmed.

My wife and I both work in a large university hospital. We thought we knew, at least in general terms, what autism was and we were devastated. I thought of children I'd seen during my medical training. They lived in institutions; they rocked back and forth, flapped their hands continually and muttered incomprehensible words, screeched when you touched them, or were just silent. In some ways, I felt as if the neurologist had told us that our son was dead.

Though my son was only three when he was diagnosed, I already had great plans for him. He was a beautiful boy, strong and healthy. His college fund was started and I knew he was bound for the Ivy League. He would play sports; do well in school. He'd become the president of his class. He would have all the advantages I never had. He would be successful and he would make me proud. Now I was told that none of that would ever happen. My dreams, at least, were dead.

For weeks, my wife and I were in shock. We didn't discuss the diagnosis with our families or friends. We stopped socializing and spent more time at home staring at our son and wondering what the future held for him and us.

At the prompting of the pediatric neurologist, we sought out an early intervention program offered by the local school district. Though he was only three, Campion attended a full day of school. There he received speech, occupational, and physical therapy.

At first, the progress was slow, and Campion fought us every day. Getting him fed, dressed, and onto the bus in the morning was an Olympian struggle. His tantrums increased as did our stress level.

My wife and I learned a lot about autism. We read books and articles. We attended lectures and sought counseling. Importantly, we met other families with autistic children. We found that we were not alone in our fears and ignorance. Our meeting others with autistic children was both a great source of comfort and practical information. We learned how to create structure at home that would calm our son's anxiety. We learned the basics of behavior modification and how to communicate with and motivate our son. It was challenging.

Autism is a term that refers to a collection of developmental disorders that affect the brain. This brain disorder affects a person's ability to communicate, form relationships with others, and respond appropriately to the external world.

But slowly, Campion's behavior improved. He began to speak a few words rather than pulling us or pointing; then he used short sentences. In those first few months after his diagnosis, I was convinced that he would never speak. This improvement was thrilling. Everyday tasks such as bathing, brushing his teeth, and getting dressed were taught. Each task was broken down into its component parts. Each part was taught slowly, sequentially, and repeated often—but he learned them. He now completes them independently and without prompting. The whole family takes pride in these triumphs.

Campion can still be a challenge at times. Autism makes him rigid in his scheduling and finicky in his choice of foods and clothing, but he continues to make progress. He enjoys playing with his trains and drawing pictures of dinosaurs. He laughs at the cartoons on TV and dances with his sisters. He's different, but loveable and loving.

My wife and I have come to realize that our grief about his diagnosis was the feeling of loss about *our* plans and *our* ambitions for him. We now have new plans and new ambitions for him. We have hope.

Campion Quinn, MD

PART 1

The Basics

What is autism?

What is the prognosis for
children with autism?

More . . .

Autism
A developmental disturbance that is characterized by an abnormal or impaired development in social communication and interaction skills and significantly restricted range of activities and interests.

Cognitive
A term that describes mental processes by which the sensory input is transformed, stored, and retrieved.

Social skills
Defined as cognitive and overt behaviors a person uses in interpersonal interactions and can range from simple nonverbal behaviors such as eye contact and head nods to the complex verbal behavior of offering a compromise that will meet everyone's needs.

1. What is autism?

Autism is a term that refers to a collection of developmental disorders that affect the brain. This brain disorder affects a person's ability to communicate, form relationships with others, and respond appropriately to the external world. People with autism have a tendency to have repetitive behaviors or interests and rigid patterns of thinking. The severity of autism varies greatly. Some people with autism can function at a relatively high level, with speech and intelligence intact. Others have serious **cognitive** impairments and language delays; some never speak.

An infant with autism may avoid eye contact, seem deaf, and abruptly stop developing language and **social skills**. It has been reported that approximately 20 percent of children with autism experience this type of neurologic "regression."

The autistic child may act as if unaware of the coming and going of others or physically attack and injure others without provocation. Infants with autism often remain fixated on a single item or activity, rock or flap their hands, seem insensitive to burns and bruises, and may even appear to purposely injure themselves.

The disorder generally becomes apparent in children by the age of three, although some children are diagnosed at older ages. Boys are three to four times more likely to have autism than girls are. When girls are afflicted with the disorder, they tend to have more severe symptoms and greater cognitive impairment.

Autism occurs in all racial, ethnic, and social groups. Though the cause of autism is unknown, a variety of factors could be associated with some forms of autism. These include infectious, metabolic, genetic, neurological, and environmental factors such as diet, exposure to toxins or medications.

A physician at Johns Hopkins Hospital named Dr. Leo Kanner studied a group of 11 developmentally delayed children in the early 1940s. Based on their characteristic self-involvement and self-stimulatory behavior, he coined the term *early infantile* autism. A group of children with similar, but milder neurologic symptoms was studied by a German scientist named Dr. Hans Asperger at about the same time as Dr. Kanner. This milder form of autism became known as **Asperger syndrome (AS)**.

2. What are the autism spectrum disorders (ASDs)?

Autism is one of a spectrum of five related neurological and developmental disorders called pervasive developmental disorders (PDDs) or **autism spectrum disorders (ASDs)**.

This group of disorders includes:

1. **Autism**—A severe form of ASD
2. **Pervasive developmental disorder–not otherwise specified (PDD–NOS)**—A diagnosis made when a child has symptoms of either of autism or Asperger's syndrome, but does not meet the specific criteria for either of them
3. **Asperger's syndrome**—A milder form of ASD
4. **Rett syndrome**—A rare, very severe neurological disorder that occurs more commonly in females

Asperger syndrome (AS)

A developmental disorder on the autism spectrum defined by impairments in communication and social development and by narrow interests and repetitive behaviors. Unlike typical autism, individuals with Asperger syndrome have no significant delay in language or cognitive development. People with Asperger syndrome have difficulty with social understanding, and their patterns of behavior are often inflexible. Language, and especially abstract language, can be hard for these people.

Autism spectrum disorders (ASDs)

A term that encompasses autism and similar disorders. More specifically, the following five disorders listed in the *DSM-IV*: autistic disorder, Asperger syndrome, pervasive developmental disorder–not otherwise specified, childhood disintegrative disorder, and Rett syndrome.

The Basics

Pervasive developmental disorders (PDDs)

These are a group of neurologic disorders of unknown cause that are marked by impairment in developmental areas such as social interaction and communication or stereotyped behavior, interests, and activities. The disorders include autistic disorder, Rett syndrome, childhood disintegrative disorder, Asperger syndrome, and pervasive developmental disorder–not otherwise specified.

Childhood disintegrative disorder (CDD)

A condition occurring in 3- and 4-year-olds characterized by a deterioration of intellectual, social, and language functioning from previously normal functioning. Children with this condition, which is sometimes misdiagnosed as autism, develop normally for a prolonged period of time, but then experience loss of social skills, bowel and bladder control, play behaviors, receptive and expressive language, motor skills, and nonverbal communication skills.

5. **Childhood disintegrative disorder (CDD)**—A rare and severe developmental disorder

This group of developmental disabilities is caused by one or more unknown abnormalities in the brain. All these disorders are characterized by varying degrees of impairment in communication skills, social interactions, and restricted, repetitive, and stereotyped patterns of behavior. These children and adults can exhibit extreme rigidity in their schedules and daily activities. They can have unusual ways of learning and paying attention. They can sometimes react abnormally to normal situations or sensations.

ASDs are more common than many better known disorders such as diabetes, spina bifida, or **Down syndrome**. ASDs occur in up to 6 out of every 1,000 children born in the United States. This is similar to the rates measured in other countries, such as the United Kingdom, Europe, and Asia. The controversy surrounding the reports of rising rates of autism will be discussed later in this book.

Characteristic behaviors of autism begin early in life, usually in the first year. The child's parents are usually the first to notice these behaviors, but not recognize them as a problem. Parents may report to the pediatrician that their child is unresponsive to verbal commands, or that he spends an inordinate amount of time playing with one toy, especially toys that spin. The parents may think the child has a hearing problem. Professionals can reliably diagnose autism by the age of three. In cases where the symptoms are pronounced, a diagnosis can be made by the age of 18 months. Some researchers claim that many children eventually may be accurately identified by the age of 1 year or even younger.

Some parents may report that their child appeared to be developing normally, that he or she was responsive, interactive, and had normal speech development, and then suddenly became quiet, didn't obey commands or want to play. This phenomenon is called "autistic regression" and for many years was controversial. Some scientists claimed that this regression was actually the inaccurate recall or "wishful thinking" of parents. However, researchers have studied family videos of children whose parents reported this phenomenon. The scientists noted that these children had normal speech patterns, object pointing and interactive playing at 12 months that was not present at 24 months of age. It is not known if autistic children who experience this regressive phenomenon are different from those autistic children who don't.

Research has shown that parents are usually correct about noticing developmental problems, although they may not realize the specific nature or degree of the problem. Therefore, when physicians and psychologists attempt to diagnose a child with autism, they will spend a lot of time asking the parents questions about the child's behavior.

The appearance of any of the warning signs of ASD is reason to have a child evaluated by a professional specializing in these disorders. The earlier the disorder is diagnosed, the sooner the child can be helped through treatment **interventions**. **Early intervention** is associated with improved behavioral outcomes.

William's comment:

Our son Liam was diagnosed at age 2 1/2. We first had suspicions when our son was about 1 1/2 years old. He wasn't responding to his name, didn't seem to understand things

Down syndrome

A genetic condition in which an individual has 47 chromosomes instead of 46; typically characterized by physical anomalies and developmental delays; the most frequently occurring chromosomal disorder.

Interventions

Types of traditional or nontraditional treatments that may be effective in reducing autistic behaviors.

Early intervention

Specific services that are provided to infants and toddlers who show signs of, or are at risk of, having a developmental delay. These services are often tailored to the specific needs of each child with the goal of furthering development. Early intervention services are often provided at no cost to children who qualify and their families.

The Basics

we said when his peers did, covered his ears at certain sounds. It wasn't as if these things were constant; they were happening intermittently over several months.

Pediatrician

A medical doctor who specializes in the treatment and care of infants, children, and adolescents.

*We called our **pediatrician** who told us to wait another 3 months and call him then for a re-evaluation. If anyone gives you that advice, fire them. Get another doctor who is more familiar with developmental delays. Nothing is lost by having your child see a developmental specialist. The best course of action with autistic kids is early intervention; therefore waiting makes no sense.*

*Within the next 3 months, others close to us suggested there might be a problem. We called a developmental pediatrician. The developmental pediatrician told us within 10 minutes of our visit with him that something was wrong. He was certain Liam was autistic. After that statement, things seemed to blur. He spoke, but we were so shell shocked that it made comprehending anything else he said impossible. He did say something about living a fulfilling life; he gave us a few phone numbers, one to our local regional center; another to a **child psychologist** who could administer further testing.*

Child psychologist

A mental health professional with a doctorate in psychology who administers tests, evaluates, and treats children's emotional disorders; cannot prescribe medication.

The following day we called him back with several questions. I asked him where on a scale of 1–10 he felt our son was (with 10 being the most severe). He answered: "around a 3 or a 4." I asked him will it get worse? He said no, where it is, is usually where it stays. Lastly, I asked him . . . I forget.

We quickly found a child psychologist who spent about 3 hours with Liam and came to the same conclusion as the developmental pediatrician.

Still not convinced, we then had several autism screening tests administered by a psychologist and the results were consistent with what the pediatrician told us in his 10-minute evaluation. We kind of figured by then that autism wasn't that hard to diagnose.

My wife Rebecca parked herself in front of the computer, got on the Web and stayed on it for what seemed like an eternity. She kept coming back to the same thing in regard to treatment: **applied behavioral analysis (ABA)**—*the only treatment with scientific data to back up its claims. We were on the ball enough to see through the "swimming with dolphins" and "talking to horses" nonsense.*

We immediately sought out an intense ABA program for him. We learned that the service providers had waiting lists anywhere from 9 to 18 months to get in. We immediately found an independent therapist and began putting together programs. By some miracle, a space opened up in one of the agencies 8 weeks later. We were in.

3. What is Asperger syndrome?

Asperger syndrome (or Asperger disorder) is a neurological disorder that may be part of the autistic spectrum of disorders. Children with Asperger syndrome have characteristic behaviors that can cause disabilities that range from mild to severe. Asperger syndrome is sometimes referred to as **high-functioning autism (HFA)** and was named for a Viennese physician, Hans Asperger. Dr. Asperger published a paper in 1944, which described a pattern of behaviors in several young boys who had normal intelligence and language development, but who also exhibited autistic-like behaviors and marked deficiencies in social and communication skills. In spite of the publication of his paper in the 1940s, it wasn't until 1994 that Asperger syndrome was added to the fourth edition of the ***Diagnostic and Statistical Manual of Mental Disorders (DSM-IV)*** and

The Basics

Applied behavioral analysis (ABA)

A system of early educational intervention first developed by Ivar Lovaas. It uses a series of trials to shape a desired behavior or response. Skills are broken down into their simplest components and then taught to the child through a system of reinforcement. It is designed to promote appropriate language and behaviors and to reduce problematic ones.

High-functioning autism (HFA)

Individuals with autism who are not cognitively impaired. Sometimes used as a synonym of Asperger syndrome.

Diagnostic and Statistical Manual (DSM-IV)

The official system for classification of psychological and psychiatric disorders prepared and published by the American Psychiatric Association.

only in the past few years has AS been recognized by professionals and parents.

Social communication

Refers to language that is used in social situations. During the school years, this refers to a child's ability to use language to interact with others in a host of situations, from entering peer groups to resolving conflicts.

Social communication deficits are a central characteristic of Asperger syndrome, although these deficits can vary in extent. Though those with the disorder show no indication of primary language impairment, their actual conversation skills are poor. Children with Asperger syndrome have problems with pragmatic responses, as well as difficulty understanding and expressing the emotional content of communication.

Vocabularies of children with Asperger syndrome may be extraordinarily rich and nuanced; on the other hand, these children can also be extremely literal and have difficulty using language in a social context.

Nonverbal

There are two types of interpersonal communication: verbal and nonverbal. Nonverbal communication includes information that is transmitted without words, through body language, gestures, facial expressions, or the use of symbols.

The *DSM-IV* gives the diagnostic criteria for Asperger syndrome as:

Qualitative impairment in social interaction, as manifested by at least two of the following:

Emotional reciprocity

An impaired or deviant response to other people's emotions; lack of modulation of behavior according to social context; and/or a weak integration of social, emotional, and communicative behaviors.

- *marked impairments in the use of multiple **nonverbal** behaviors such as eye-to-eye gaze, facial expression, body postures, and gestures to regulate social interaction*
- *failure to develop peer relationships appropriate to developmental level*
- *a lack of spontaneous seeking to share enjoyment, interests, or achievements with other people (e.g., by a lack of showing, bringing, or pointing out objects of interest to other people)*
- *lack of social or **emotional reciprocity***

Restricted repetitive and stereotyped patterns of behavior, interests, and activities, as manifested by at least one of the following:

- *encompassing preoccupation with one or more stereotyped and restricted patterns of interest that is abnormal either in intensity or focus*
- *apparently inflexible adherence to specific, nonfunctional routines or rituals*
- *stereotyped and repetitive motor mannerisms (e.g., hand or finger flapping or twisting or complex whole-body movements)*
- *persistent preoccupation with parts of objects*
- *The disturbance causes clinically significant impairment in social, occupational, or other important areas of functioning.*

Language:

There is no clinically significant general delay in language (e.g., single words used by age 2 years, communicative phrases used by age 3 years).

Cognitive Development:

*There is no clinically significant delay in **cognitive development** or in the development of age-appropriate self-help skills, adaptive behavior (other than social interaction), and curiosity about the environment in childhood; that is, they have normal or high intelligence levels.*

Does not meet other diagnostic criteria:

*Criteria are not met for another specific pervasive developmental disorder or **schizophrenia**.*

The Basics

Cognitive development

The development of the functions of the brain including perception, memory, imagination, and use of language.

Schizophrenia

A psychotic disorder characterized by loss of contact with the environment, by noticeable deterioration in the level of functioning in everyday life, and by disintegration of personality expressed as disorder of feeling, thought (as in hallucinations and delusions), and conduct.

4. How can you tell autism from Asperger syndrome?

According to the American Academy of Child and Adolescent Psychiatry (AACAP), Asperger syndrome is characterized by problems with behavior and development of social skills. Because of similarities to symptoms of autism, some practitioners feel that children with these symptoms need careful evaluation and that they may benefit from different types of therapies. AACAP draws the following similarities and differences between autism and Asperger syndrome:

- Asperger syndrome appears to have a somewhat later onset than autistic disorder or at least to be recognized later.
- A child with Asperger syndrome typically functions at a higher level than a child with autism does.
- It is common for a child with Asperger syndrome to have normal to above-normal intelligence.
- Although children with Asperger syndrome may have unusual speech patterns, there is usually no delay in language development.
- In contrast to autistic disorder, there are no clinically significant delays in cognitive development or in the development of age-appropriate self-help skills, adaptive behavior, and curiosity about the environment in childhood.
- Children with Asperger syndrome may have trouble interacting with children their age. They are often loners and may show behavior that some people may consider eccentric.
- Many children with Asperger syndrome have problems with muscular coordination and fine motor skills.

Like autism, a specific cause for Asperger syndrome is not yet known, although there may be a tendency for the condition to run in families.

According to the AACAP, like autism, a specific cause for Asperger syndrome is not yet known, although there may be a tendency for the condition to run in families. This may suggest a genetic link, though recent genetic studies have not revealed an "Asperger gene." The AACAP states that children with Asperger syndrome are at a higher risk for psychiatric problems including depression, **attention deficit hyperactivity disorder (ADHD)**, schizophrenia, and **obsessive-compulsive disorder (OCD)** than autistic children. Unlike autistic children, many children with Asperger syndrome finish high school and attend college and can develop healthy relationships outside of their family.

In personal experience, children with autism who have relatively mild symptoms and high IQs are variously referred to by different clinicians as having autism, high-functioning autism, mild autism, and Asperger disorder. This causes much confusion for parents and professionals and implies that these diagnoses represent separate and distinct disorders differing in clinically meaningful ways and requiring different treatments, which may not be the case.

5. What is pervasive developmental disorder–not otherwise specified?

Pervasive developmental disorder–not otherwise specified (PDD–NOS) is a **developmental disability** that shares many characteristics with autism.

Often doctors will simply use the shorthand "PDD" when referring to PDD–NOS, but this is incorrect. The term PDD refers to the class of conditions to

Attention deficit hyperactivity disorder (ADHD)

A disorder of childhood and adolescence characterized by lack of impulse control, inability to concentrate, and hyperactivity. A particular symptom complex with core symptoms including developmentally inappropriate degrees of attention, cognitive disorganization, distractibility, impulsivity, and hyperactivity, all of which vary in different situations and at different times. Also called *attention deficit disorder (ADD)*.

Obsessive-compulsive disorder (OCD)

Having a tendency to perform certain repetitive acts or ritualistic behavior to relieve anxiety.

The Basics

Pervasive developmental disorder–not otherwise specified (PDD–NOS)

One of the five diagnoses in the autistic spectrum of diseases. The diagnosis of PDD–NOS is used when there is severe impairment in social interaction and verbal and nonverbal communication skills or when stereotyped behavior, interests, and activities are present, but symptoms do not meet the criteria for other autistic disorders.

Developmental disability (DD)

A disability of a person manifested before the age of 22 and expected to continue indefinitely. Attributable to mental retardation, cerebral palsy, epilepsy, autism, brain injury, or another neurological condition closely related to mental retardation or requiring treatment similar to that required for mental retardation; results in substantial functional limitations in three or more major areas of life activity.

which autism belongs. PDD is therefore not itself a **diagnosis** but a group of diagnoses, while PDD–NOS is a diagnosis.

PDD–NOS is probably the most commonly diagnosed condition within the ASD and is sometimes referred to as "atypical personality development," "atypical PDD," or "**atypical autism.**"

Children are diagnosed with PDD–NOS when they exhibit significant difficulties in the areas of social interaction, verbal communication (speech), nonverbal communication (gesture; eye contact), and play, but are too social to be considered fully autistic or any of the other explicitly defined PDDs, such as Rett syndrome or childhood disintegrative disorder. This is why PDD–NOS is sometimes considered a "subthreshold" condition. Put another way, a diagnosis of autistic disorder is made when an individual displays 6 or more of 12 symptoms listed across three major areas: social interaction, communication, and behavior. However, when children display many of these behaviors but do not meet the full criteria for autistic disorder, they may receive a diagnosis of PDD–NOS.

Though the symptoms of PDD–NOS are usually manifest by the age of 3 years, studies have demonstrated that these children are usually diagnosed later and receive treatment later than other autistic children. This delay results from the confusion with the diagnosis, the comparatively less-severe behavioral symptoms, and that intellectual deficits are less common.

It should be emphasized that this subthreshold category is defined by what symptoms the child lacks from the diagnosis of autism, rather than what symptoms the child has. No specific guidelines for diagnosis are provided. This lack of clear criteria for this large and diverse group of children presents problems for research on this condition.

6. What is Rett syndrome?

Rett syndrome is a disorder of the nervous system that has some of the same characteristics as autism. Both diseases strike at an early age, and a loss of language and social interaction are common in both. Like autism, children suffering from Rett syndrome will avoid eye contact, have a diminished ability to express feelings, and will exhibit purposeless hand movements such as flapping, wringing, or waving. Seizures are common in both diseases, and neither has a known cure.

Despite the similarities, Rett syndrome and autism are distinct diseases with many differences that distinguish them. Autism is a disease with a male predominance, while Rett syndrome is found in females almost exclusively. The neurologic deficits of autism remain stable; however, Rett syndrome is a progressive neurological disorder, whose symptoms worsen as the child gets older. Autistic children are often first diagnosed because of speech and social interaction, though the first symptom noticed in children with Rett syndrome is loss of muscle tone (called **hypotonia** by physicians.)

Like autism, Rett syndrome knows no geographic, racial, or social boundaries. Fewer then 1 percent of Rett cases have a familial inheritance pattern; that is, very few cases are found in families who have relatives with Rett syndrome.

The Basics

Diagnosis
Identification of a disease, disorder, or syndrome through a method of consistent analysis.

Atypical autism
A general term for conditions that are close to but don't quite fit the set of conditions for autism or other specific conditions. This condition is also referred to as pervasive developmental disorder—not otherwise specified or PDD–NOS.

Hypotonia
Decreased muscle tone.

Gene

Originally defined as the physical unit of heredity, it is probably best defined as the unit of inheritance that occupies a specific locus on a chromosome, the existence of which can be confirmed by the occurrence of different allelic forms. Genes are formed from DNA, carried on the chromosomes, and are responsible for the inherited characteristics that distinguish one individual from another. Each human individual has an estimated 100,000 separate genes.

Chromosome

Structure in the cell nucleus that bears an individual's genetic information.

Rett syndrome is known to be associated with mutations in the **gene** MECP2 located on the X **chromosome**. It is not known if this gene mutation causes Rett syndrome or is just a marker for the disease. Nevertheless, the discovery of the MECP2 gene has made possible the development of a blood test for Rett syndrome. Approximately 85 percent of all patients diagnosed with Rett syndrome also test positive for an MECP2 mutation. This does not mean that the remaining 15 percent do not have Rett syndrome. Although testing positive for a mutation confirms the diagnosis, it is not required. The diagnosis of the disorder, however, is still based on symptoms and clinical history. It is possible that mutations exist in an area of MECP2 that has not yet been sequenced or perhaps other genes contribute to Rett syndrome. No blood test yet exists for the diagnosis of autism.

The following criteria are used for making a clinical diagnosis of Rett syndrome. Please keep in mind that Rett syndrome is a spectrum disorder like autism. Not all the symptoms are seen in every patient and the severity of a symptom may vary widely from patient to patient.

Diagnostic Criteria

- Period of apparent normal development until 6–18 months
- Regression (in other words, a change from normal early development into impaired abilities)
- Diminished ability to express feelings
- Avoidance of eye contact
- Grinding teeth
- Loss of verbal language
- Purposeful hand use replaced by stereotypical hand movements such as flapping or waving

- Normal head circumference at birth followed by slowing of the rate of head growth
- If able to walk, gait is usually wide-based and stiff-legged
- Shakiness of torso and/or limbs, especially when upset
- Growth retardation and decreased body fat and muscle mass

Although some individuals with Rett syndrome die at a young age, the majority live into adulthood. Autism, on the other hand, is not associated with a reduced life span.

7. What is childhood disintegrative disorder?

Childhood disintegrative disorder (CDD) is a neurological condition with similarities to autism. This condition can be differentiated from autism by the pattern of onset, its course, and outcome.

With CDD, children develop a condition that resembles autism, but only after a relatively prolonged period of normal neurological and behavioral development (usually 2 to 4 years) followed by extensive and pronounced neurological losses involving motor, language, and social skills. Accompanying the motor and language losses, there is a loss of interest in social interaction and a general loss of interest in the environment. The loss of skills such as vocabulary is more dramatic in CDD than it is in classical autism—this helps to distinguish the two diseases. As CDD progresses, often toileting and self-care abilities are lost, the child may develop seizures, and IQs are very low. The child comes to look profoundly autistic in his or her behaviors, but their disease does not

Childhood disintegrative disorder (CDD) is a neurological condition with similarities to autism. This condition can be differentiated from autism by the pattern of onset, its course, and outcome.

The Basics

progress the same as autism. As with autism, children who suffer from this condition are at increased risk for seizures. The current available data suggest that the **prognosis** for CDD is generally worse than that for autism.

CDD was first described in 1908 by an educator in Vienna, Theodore Heller, who called it *dementia infantalis*. CDD characteristics were recognized many years before autism was described. Despite this, CDD has only recently been recognized officially and was frequently misdiagnosed in the past.

CDD is a rare condition. Based on four surveys, an estimate found fewer than 2 children per 100,000 with ASD who could be classified as having CDD. Put another way, strictly defined autism is approximately 10 times more common than CDD. More boys are affected with CDD than girls.

The **etiology** is unknown but several lines of evidence suggest that CDD arises as a result of some form of central nervous system pathology; the specific cause, however, is unknown. There is no known cure.

8. What is the prognosis of children with autism?

Autism is a life-long disorder. Predicting an autistic child's future, in regards to social abilities, scholastic achievement, and vocational potential, is difficult even for experts without a full neurological assessment and several months or years of observations. Experts look for certain predictors of future abilities, such as intelligence, verbal ability, and socialization.

The most important prognostic factor is the IQ of the child. In addition, the degree of social interaction impairment and lack of appropriate communication early on correlate with the severity of the outcome. The most accurate predictor of outcome, however, is the progression over a period of about 1 year from early diagnosis. Those with mild behavioral symptoms and few autistic features may do remarkably well.

Once established, the neurologic deficits of autism neither improve nor worsen during a child's life. However, with treatment, the disabilities of autism, such as speech impairment and social interaction, can be improved in many children. This is especially true when the child is diagnosed early and treated early. Early intervention that includes behavioral modification and speech therapy has been shown to improve outcomes in autistic children. In fact, some children with autism who receive proper treatment and social support grow up to lead normal or near-normal lives. The Autism Society of America reports that many people with autism enjoy their lives and contribute to their communities.

The majority of children, unfortunately, will require supervision and support of various amounts throughout their lives. The amount of supervision and social support required depends on the extent of their disabilities.

Epilepsy is a problem with up to one third of children with autism. Children whose language skills regress early in life, usually before the age of 3, appear to be at higher risk of developing epilepsy or seizure-like brain activity.

Epilepsy
A neurological disorder that can lead to convulsions, partial and full loss of consciousness, and absences. It occurs more frequently in autistic people and their families than in the general population.

Neuropsychiatric disorders are also associated with autism. During adolescence, some children with autism may become depressed or experience behavioral problems. Parents of these children should be ready to adjust treatment for their child as needed.

According to the **National Institutes of Health (NIH)**, people with autism have normal life expectancies.

William's comment:

We've seen older children who are now mainstreamed in school, and even referred to as "indistinguishable" and have had their services "faded." Granted, it's not all the kids, but there are some who do remarkably well with ABA.

*Our son has been getting ABA-based services for around 1 year now. Although we don't know what the future holds, we have seen tremendous progress in that time. His tantrums are a fraction of what they were a year before. His **self-stimulatory behavior (stims)** seem to have decreased also. He even has promising moments of acknowledging peers, and his speech has come so far from where it was.*

Watching him make strides is very rewarding for us.

9. Are there other diseases that have the same symptoms of autism?

When a child is brought to the pediatrician and the parents report that their child is not speaking yet, the pediatrician considers several possible diagnoses, one of which is autism. Because several conditions may be confused with autism, the pediatrician must be careful when making the final determination about a child's disorder and its management. Any condition that may be associated with language delay, especially those that are treatable, must be considered.

National Institutes of Health (NIH)

Located in Bethesda, Maryland, it is the largest governmental medical research center. It is part of the U.S. Department of Health and Human Services. It is composed of 27 separate institutes and is charged with the mission to improve the health of the people of the United States

Self-stimulatory behaviors (stims)

This is the name given to the purposeless repetitive actions that some autistic people feel compelled to do. Examples are hand flapping, spinning, toe walking, and so forth.

- **Hearing loss**: Every child with a language delay must have a hearing test. Confusion is common because deaf children can mimic autistic symptoms. For example, a deaf child may present with "pervasive ignoring," production of unusual sounds, and poor socialization because he or she is unable to hear the sounds or speech around him. He may exhibit poor eye contact because he can't coordinate his eyes to the direction of the sound. Frustration in a lack of ability to communicate may result in temper tantrums. Children with deafness who are treated early and appropriately will make a rapid recovery of lost language. For this reason, a hearing test is always important to obtain in a child with a speech delay (even if the parents think their child can hear) because the hearing loss may be partial or selective to different frequencies.

Because several conditions may be confused with autism, the pediatrician must be careful when making the final determination about a child's disorder and its management.

The Basics

William's comment:

We had to jump through the hoop of having our child undergo a hearing test, even though everyone knew that wasn't the problem.

- **Mental retardation**: Another condition that may mimic autism is mental retardation. It may present with speech delay, and, if severe enough, self-stimulatory behaviors and other autistic characteristics may be associated. A common cause of mental retardation is Down syndrome. This occurs in approximately 1 in 800 births. Although rare, some scientific studies have found subjects with Down syndrome and autism. Although autism is rare in persons with Down syndrome, it should be considered in the range of diagnostic possibilities for persons with this syndrome. When autism affects a child with Down syndrome, the effects are quite severe and, therefore, the autism condition must be the priority condition.

- **Acquired epileptiform aphasia (also known as Landau-Kleffner syndrome)**: **Landau-Kleffner syndrome** is a rare form of childhood epilepsy that is associated with a severe language disorder. The cause of Landau-Kleffner syndrome is unknown. The syndrome occurs in young children, mostly older than 3 years of age but occasionally younger. They develop seizure activity and have associated **autistic regression** and loss of acquired speech. Because of that, it is recommended that physicians obtain an EEG (sleep deprived or 24-hour recording) on those autistic children who have a history of loss of acquired speech and behavioral regression. The Landau-Kleffner syndrome can be successfully treated with antiepileptic drugs and ACTH.

- **Fragile X syndrome**: Fragile X syndrome is one of the most common causes of genetically inherited mental retardation. Mental impairment can range from subtle learning disabilities and a normal IQ to severe cognitive or intellectual challenges. Other symptoms often include unique physical characteristics (e.g., long face with a prominent jaw and large prominent ears), behavioral deficits, and delays in speech and language development that mimic autistic-like behavior. The syndrome is called "fragile X" because there exists a fragile site or gap at the end of the long arm of the X chromosome in lymphocytes of affected patients. Carrier females typically have a 30 to 40 percent chance of giving birth to a retarded male and a 15 to 20 percent chance of having a retarded female. Further, there frequently exists a maternal family history for a relative with mental retardation or developmental and learning disabilities. Most studies have dealt with recognition of this syndrome in older children and young adults, but many of the physical features, behavioral characteristics, and family history features are apparent earlier. Experts suggest that all children with autism should be tested for fragile X syndrome.

- **Childhood schizophrenia**: This rare disorder can mimic autism. Childhood schizophrenia occurs in less than 1 in 10,000 births and affects slightly more males than females. This condition usually develops after 5 years of age and is associated with a higher IQ score (more than 70) than what is found with autism. The typical patterns of behavior before a formal diagnosis include problems with attention and conduct, social withdrawal, and hypersensitivity to sounds, noises, and textures. More than 80 percent of children have auditory hallucinations; 50 percent have delusional beliefs.

- **Tuberous sclerosis**: This affects approximately 1 in 10,000 people and is characterized by abnormal tissue growth or benign tumors in the brain and other organs such as the skin, kidneys, eyes, heart, and lungs. Autistic-like symptoms were first described in patients with **tuberous sclerosis** a decade before Kanner's classic delineation of infantile autism. These early noted symptoms include stereotypes, absent or abnormal speech, withdrawal, and impaired interactions. Today, the Tuberous Sclerosis Society suggests that approximately 60 percent of its membership have autism or autistic-like behavior or symptoms.

- **Williams syndrome**: Williams syndrome is a rare genetic condition (estimated to occur in 1 in 20,000 births) that causes medical and developmental problems. Williams syndrome was first recognized as a distinct entity in 1961. It is present at birth and affects males and females equally. It can occur

Tuberous sclerosis

A neurocutaneous disorder characterized by mental retardation, seizures, skin lesions, and intracranial lesions. It is caused by a dominant gene and occurs in 1 in 7,000 births.

Developmental delays

A term used to describe the development of children who have not reached various milestones in the time frame that is typical for children of his or her chronological age; may occur in one or more areas of functioning.

Perseveration

This refers to a persistent and often purposeless repetition of speech or movement.

Congenital

Any trait or condition that exists from birth.

in all ethnic groups and has been identified in countries throughout the world. It is caused, in most cases, by a deletion in one of the chromosomes that contain the gene for the protein elastin. People with Williams syndrome often show a distinctive cognitive profile. They have some degree of intellectual handicap as well as **developmental delays** in their "milestones" such as walking, talking, and toilet training. Children with Williams syndrome have some typical autistic traits including distractibility. The distractibility seems to get worse in mid-childhood, but appears to get better as the children get older. Other "autistic traits" common in Williams syndrome include extreme hearing sensitivity, obsessive worrying, **perseveration**, repetitive purposeless movements, difficulties relating to peers, and body rocking. Despite these similarities, children with Williams can be distinguished from autistic children because of other characteristics. These characteristics include:

- A very friendly and endearing personality
- Strong expressive language skills
- They are typically unafraid of strangers.
- They demonstrate a greater interest in contact with adults than with their peers.

Relations between Williams syndrome and autism have not yet been widely studied.

- **Cornelia de Lange syndrome:** Cornelia de Lange syndrome (CDLS) is a multiple **congenital** anomaly syndrome. The exact incidence is unclear, but it is thought to be between 1 in 10,000 and 1 in 30,000 live births. The syndrome is characterized by the following:
  - a distinctive facial appearance, including a small head size, eyebrows that meet at the mid-

line, long eyelashes, short up-turned nose, and thin down-turned lips

- prenatal and postnatal growth deficiency (low birth weight)
- feeding difficulties
- delays in reaching typical developmental milestones (especially in receptive and expressive language)
- behavioral problems (heightened sensitivity to touch; behavioral difficulties including hyperactivity, short attention span, oppositional and repetitive behavior, and **self-injurious behavior [SIB]**)
- Physical malformations involving the arms and hands

Because these behavioral characteristics are similar in many ways to those present in individuals with autism, "autistic-like behaviors" are listed as an associated complication for individuals with Cornelia de Lange syndrome.

10. Do autistic children commonly suffer from other illnesses?

Individuals with autism often have symptoms of various mental disorders that occur at the same time. These disorders include: ADHD, psychoses, depressive disorders, tics, **Tourette's syndrome**, obsessive-compulsive disorder, and other anxiety disorders. About one third of children and adolescents with autism develop seizures.

Sensory problems. When children's perceptions are accurate, they can learn from what they see, feel, or

---

Self-injurious behavior (SIB)

Self-inflicted bodily harm; harm done to the self by an individual. Individuals with an autistic spectrum disorder are often prone to self-injurious behavior.

Tourette's syndrome

An inherited, neurological disorder characterized by repeated and involuntary body movements (tics) and uncontrollable vocal sounds. In a minority of cases, the vocalizations can include socially inappropriate words and phrases; this is called coprolalia. These outbursts are neither intentional nor purposeful. Involuntary symptoms can include eye blinking, repeated throat clearing or sniffing, arm thrusting, kicking movements, shoulder shrugging, or jumping. The disturbance causes marked distress or significant impairment in social, occupational, or other important areas of functioning.

The Basics

Many autistic children are highly attuned or even painfully sensitive to certain sounds, textures, tastes, and smells.

hear. On the other hand, if sensory information is faulty, the child's experiences of the world can be confusing. Many autistic children are highly attuned or even painfully sensitive to certain sounds, textures, tastes, and smells. Some children find the feel of clothes touching their skin almost unbearable. Some sounds—a vacuum cleaner, a ringing telephone, a sudden storm, even the sound of waves lapping the shoreline—will cause these children to cover their ears and scream.

In autism, the brain seems unable to balance the senses appropriately. Some autistic children are oblivious to extreme cold or pain. An autistic child may fall and break an arm, yet never cry. Another may bash his or her head against a wall and not wince, but a light touch may make the child scream with alarm.

Mental retardation. Many children with autism have some degree of mental impairment. When tested, some areas of ability may be normal, while others may be especially weak. For example, a child with autism may do well on the parts of the test that measure visual skills but earn low scores on the language subtests.

Seizures. One in four children with autism develops seizures, often starting in either early childhood or adolescence. Seizures, caused by abnormal electrical activity in the brain, can produce a temporary loss of consciousness (a "blackout"), a body convulsion, unusual movements, or staring spells. Sometimes a contributing factor is a lack of sleep or a high fever. An **electroencephalogram (EEG)** can help confirm the seizure's presence.

Electroencephalogram (EEG)

A test that uses electrodes placed on the scalp to record electrical brain activity. It is often used to diagnose seizure disorders or to look for abnormal brain wave patterns.

In most cases, seizures can be controlled by a number of medicines called *anticonvulsants*. The dosage of the medication is adjusted carefully so that the least possible amount of medication will be used to be effective.

Fragile X syndrome. This disorder is the most common inherited form of mental retardation. It was so named because one part of the X chromosome has a defective piece that appears pinched and fragile when under a microscope. Fragile X syndrome affects about 2 to 5 percent of people with autism. It is important to have a child with autism checked for fragile X, especially if the parents are considering having another child. For an unknown reason, if a child with autism also has fragile X syndrome, there is a one-in-two chance that boys born to the same parents will have the syndrome. Other members of the family who may be contemplating having a child may also wish to be checked for the syndrome.

Tuberous sclerosis. Tuberous sclerosis is a rare genetic disorder that causes benign tumors to grow in the brain as well as in other vital organs. It has a consistently strong association with autism. One to 4 percent of people with autism also have tuberous sclerosis.

11. Is there an association between autism and Tourette's syndrome?

Tourette's syndrome is an inherited neurological disorder. Its symptoms begin in early childhood and are often accompanied by obsessive-compulsive behaviors. Patients suffering from Tourette's syndrome exhibit repeated and involuntary body movements (tics) and uncontrollable vocal sounds. While Tourette's syndrome is commonly associated with uncontrolled vocalizations of socially inappropriate words and phrases (**coprolalia**), this occurs in only a minority of cases. For some, the involuntary and compulsive repeated words,

Coprolalia

The involuntary uttering of vulgar or obscene words.

The Basics

29

phrases, or sounds are so severe that it makes communication impossible. The involuntary body movements can range from the innocuous, such as eye blinking or repeated throat clearing or sniffing, to more noticeable and disturbing movements such as arm thrusting, kicking movements, shoulder shrugging, or jumping.

The commonalities of stereotyped motor movements, the repetition of words and phrases, and other mannerisms have suggested an association between autism and Tourette's syndrome, which may include a possible common neurochemical abnormality. In fact, Tourette's syndrome occurs in autistic children more commonly than in the general population—up to 30 percent in some studies.

Making the diagnosis of Tourette's syndrome in an autistic child can be difficult. The characteristic behaviors of Tourette's syndrome can be mistaken autistic behaviors. For example, autistic children may exhibit self-stimulatory behaviors that resemble tics or they may perseverate sounds or words that can be mistaken for the vocal tics of Tourette's. Diagnosis for Tourette's is often delayed for several other reasons that include:

- The symptoms of Tourette's syndrome are variable and inconsistent. The symptoms that the parents observe at home can be different from those that the doctor sees when examining the child.
- Many physicians are unfamiliar with the disorder. They may dismiss the tics and vocalizations as "part of autism."
- There is no laboratory or radiologic study that can diagnose Tourette's syndrome. Instead, doctors must rely on the history of the person's symptoms.

The main criterion for a Tourette's diagnosis is the presence of both types of tics—movement and vocal—for at least a year. Attempts at limiting the tics through behavioral modification may actually increase them.

12. What are some of the common myths about autism?

Autism is puzzling disease. There is no known cause and no known cure. It strikes one child in a family and leaves another alone. It is profoundly disabling in one child and difficult to notice in another. This mystery has given rise to many myths and misconceptions about the disease. These generalizations are popularized in books and movies but are rarely appropriate. Those interested enough to investigate will learn that autistic people are as unique in their behaviors and affect as nonautistic people. The list of symptoms and behaviors associated with autism is long; each affected person expresses his or her own combination of these behaviors. Because these beliefs are widely held, it may be instructive to review some of these common myths, along with their accompanying realities.

Myth: Autism is a very rare developmental disorder.
Reality: Autism occurs in about 1 in 160 births. Autism is found all through the world in families of all racial, ethnic, and social backgrounds.

Myth: Only boys suffer from autism.
Reality: Although autism is four times more common among boys than girls, many girls are diagnosed on the autism spectrum and suffer from many symptoms of autism.

Myth: All autistic people must eventually be institutionalized.

Reality: Most autistic people live at home with their families or in group homes as they get older. Only a minority of people with autism require institutionalization. Those that are institutionalized often have severe mental retardation or other physical or neurological disabilities along with their diagnosis of autism.

Myth: Autistic people never want to be touched.

Reality: While some autistic people are **hypersensitive** to tactile stimuli (i.e., being touched or touching other things), many are fine with being touched, hugged, playing contact sports, or being examined by a physician.

Myth: Autistic people are often intellectually or musically gifted. They are capable of learning a new language in a few days, memorizing encyclopedias, or multiplying large numbers in their heads.

Reality: Approximately 70–80 percent of children with autism have IQs below average. Many are **mentally retarded (MR)**. The remainder of autistics have average or above average IQs. Very few autistic people possess remarkable mathematical skills or musical abilities. These types of gifted autistic people were called idiot savants in the past. Idiot savant is now considered a pejorative term. **Autistic savant** is the preferred term currently.

William's comment:

Describing the average autistic child as "gifted" is a stretch, certainly. However, Liam does seem to have an ear for music and can carry a tune. He does sight read and has an unusually retentive memory. Right now, at age 3 years 7 months, he's starting to read phonetically.

Hypersensitive

Excessive sensitivity to sensations or stimuli.

Mentally retarded (MR)

A person with a low cognitive ability or low IQ.

Autistic savants

Autistic individuals who display incredible aptitude for one or two skills (e.g., amazing musical or art ability).

Myth: Autism is caused by cold, distant, or abusive mothering.

Reality: Autism is a biologically caused brain disorder. While the cause of autism remains elusive, this often-quoted theory by Freud is as wrong as it is harmful. Thankfully, it has been out of favor for many years. Freud's theory is also called the "ice mother" or "**refrigerator mother**" theory.

William's comment:

"Poppycock!" Our kid got enough love to move a mountain.

Myth: Autistic children are insensitive to pain.

Reality: Although a few severely autistic may not appear to feel pain, most children react normally to painful stimuli.

Myth: Most children with autism never learn to talk.

Reality: Between 40 percent and 50 percent of children with autism have little or no language skills; this condition is often associated with severe mental retardation. However, if autistic children are identified early and undergo intensive speech therapy, as many as three quarters of autistic children are able to talk.

William's comment:

At diagnosis, Liam had very limited speech for his age. Over the past year, he has shown considerable improvement. He's not on par with his peers, but is making strides as far as fluency and expanding his vocabulary.

Myth: Children with autism never make eye contact.

Reality: Many children with autism establish eye contact. It may be less than or different from the typical child, but they do look at people, smile, and express many other wonderful nonverbal communications.

The Basics

Refrigerator mother

A phrase, in Freudian psychological theory, that was used to describe mothers who acted coldly toward their children. This behavior was once erroneously thought to be the cause of (infantile) autism.

If autistic children are identified early and undergo intensive speech therapy, as many as three quarters of autistic children are able to talk.

William's comment:

Liam's eye contact is less than a typical kid.

Myth: Autism is caused by vaccinations.
Reality: Autistic symptoms usually appear in the first two to three years of life, at a time when children are receiving many immunizations. The appearance of autistic symptoms coincident with vaccinations has led many to theorize that autism is caused by vaccinations. However, after many rigorous scientific studies, no **causal relationship** has been found.

William's comment:

We don't feel that the vaccinations had anything to do with Liam's diagnosis. We are vaccinating our daughter as well.

Myth: Autistic children show no emotion.
Reality: Autistic children can be emotionally withdrawn and may be unable to understand the emotions of others. However, they commonly exhibit love and affection, anticipation, and surprise and desire, as well as fear and anxiety. Their ability to express these emotions may be limited.

Myth: Children with autism are completely cut off from human relationships.
Reality: Autistic people may have few and atypical social relationships, but they have relationships nonetheless. Their difficulty with communication and empathy make it difficult to create friendships. However, autistic children are loveable and respond to love and affection. For example, a young child with autism may feel love and attachment for their mother and father, but still dislike being touched by them. They may develop

Causal relationship
A correlation between two variables where a change in the first variable causes a change in the second.

friendly relationships with teachers and classmates and miss them during summer vacations.

William's comment:

Liam isn't crazy about his baby sister, but we're not sure how much of this has to do with his diagnosis.

Myth: Autism is caused by chemical imbalances or allergies that can be cured by special diets or nutritional supplements.

Reality: While these theories have undeniable appeal, no credible scientific evidence exists to support the theory that autism is caused by vitamin or other nutritional deficiency nor is there evidence that diet or nutritional supplements can cure autism. Children with autism certainly can have food allergies, toxic exposures, and nutritional deficiencies and correcting these problems can help such a child to be healthier, but they won't cure autism.

Myth: Autistic people are always helpless and dependent, unable to live alone or contribute to society.

Reality: Autism is a disease with a spectrum of **disability** that ranges from nonverbal, severely retarded people completely dependent on others for their care, to those with better than average IQs and marketable skills who are able to live independently.

William's comment:

We have every reason to believe that our son will lead a very fulfilling life. He might not be throwing for 400 yards and five touchdowns on Saturday afternoons or be class president, but then again, neither will a lot of other parents' kids who are deemed "typical."

Disability
A personal limitation or challenge that represents a substantial disadvantage when attempting to function in society; should be considered within the context of the environment, personal factors, and the need for individualized supports.

PART II

Diagnosing Autism

Are there risk factors for autism?

What are some symptoms a parent should look for?

How do doctors diagnose autism?

More . . .

13. Are there risk factors for autism?

Many studies have sought to identify risk factors for autism with the hope that finding the risk factor could lead to finding a cause of autism, measures to prevent autism, or at least help to identify autistic children earlier than now is possible. While studies have found some associations, none has been identified as "causative." Researchers in one study examined the medical records of nearly 700 autistic children and their parents. This data came from Denmark's national health care system, which has records on virtually all Danish children diagnosed with autism. The study evaluated every child diagnosed with autism between 1968 and 2000. Each of the nearly 700 autistic children was compared with 25 kids without autism.

The researchers looked for issues such as medical problems the mothers may have had during pregnancy, difficulties during the birth of the child, history of mental disorders among the parents, and any illnesses the child had between birth and the diagnosis of autism.

Another group of researchers noted that head size at birth among the autistic children was smaller, on average, than the children who did not develop autism.

Researchers found that parental psychiatric histories prior to the child's diagnosis of autism had the highest association with autism. When considering all the risks, parental psychiatric history increases the risk of an autism diagnosis by three- to fourfold.

Another group of researchers noted that head size at birth among the autistic children was smaller, on average, than the children who did not develop autism. However, during the first year of life, these children experienced sudden and excessive brain growth such that their brains were larger than all but 15 percent of all measured children. This excessive growth in head size occurred well before the onset of behavioral symptoms.

These researchers went on to report that the "degree, rate, and/or duration" of the excessive brain growth may be predictive of the severity of later symptoms of autism.

The following is a list of conditions that occur more commonly in autistic children than in typical children:

- Delivery-associated risk factors:
  - breech presentation of the baby
  - low Apgar score, an index used to evaluate the condition of a newborn 5 minutes after birth
  - premature birth: (a birth before 35 weeks of pregnancy)
- Parental history of mental illness:
  - schizophrenia-like **psychosis**
  - affective disorder, which includes some psychoses, depression, and bipolar disorder
- Childhood developmental history:
  - rapid and excessive growth in head size during the first year of life

No associations have been found between autism and:

- infant weight
- number of previous babies born to the mother
- number of doctor visits before pregnancy
- parental age at time of birth of child
- socioeconomic status

Psychosis

A mental and behavioral disorder causing gross distortion or disorganization of a person's mental capacity, affective response, and capacity to recognize reality.

Diagnosing Autism

14. What are some of the symptoms of autism a parent should look for?

The diagnosis of autism covers a wide range of behaviors and abilities. No two people with autism have exactly the same symptoms or disease intensity. Autistic symptoms occur in various combinations; each can range from mild to severe. While a symptom might be mild in one person, in another it might be so severe that it overwhelms their personality or behavior. The following are examples of the common types of problems and behaviors a person with an ASD might exhibit.

Social skills. People with autism might not interact with others the way most people do or they might not be interested in other people at all. Autistic children:

- may resist cuddling by their parents
- may appear indifferent to the goings-on in their environment
- display a lack of interest in toys
- may be so unresponsive to others that they appear to be deaf
- tend not make eye contact and may be content to be alone
- as they grow older, they might appear to lack empathy or have trouble understanding other people's feelings such as pain or sorrow or talking about their own feelings
- may fail to establish friendships with children the same age
- may show a lack of interest in sharing enjoyment, interests, or achievements with other people

Speech, language, and communication. An impaired ability to communicate is one of the hallmarks of autism.

- The content of their speech may be limited to a few subjects or a just a few words. In fact, about 40 percent of children with autism do not speak at all.
- Others have **echolalia**. *Echolalia* is the medical term for an involuntary and meaningless repetition of

Echolalia

Repetitive words or phrases that autistics may say sometimes hours after the event. Delayed echolalia can occur days or weeks after hearing the word or phrase. Sometimes this will just be an echoed word. Some autistics will mimic whole sentences or even conversations; they may even use convincing accents and the voices of other people.

what has been said. People with echolalia may repeat a word, phrase, or entire sentences. For example, if somebody said to a person with echolalia, "It sure is a very nice day today." They would respond, "It sure is a very nice day today." An autistic child may repeat a television ad or part of a song heard sometime in the past. Their voices might sound flat, lacking inflection or tonal range. They may speak too loudly or too softly and it might seem like they cannot control the volume of their voice.

- Difficulties with conversation are another problem for the autistic. This might include having problems initiating a conversation. Also, people with autism have difficulties continuing a conversation once it has begun. While some people with autism may speak well and have a command of a certain subject matter, they may not understand the give-and-take nature of a conversation and will speak continuously.

- Nonverbal communication is another issue. People with autism might not understand gestures such as waving goodbye or extending a hand to shake. They tend to make poor use of body language, such as eye contact or facial expressions, as a means of nonverbal communication.

- Pronouns appear to present a difficulty. They might say "I" when they mean "you" or vice versa.

- Children with autism do not seem to understand social cues; therefore, social appropriateness can present a problem. They may stand too close to the people they are talking to, may hug or kiss strangers, or might stick with one topic of conversation for too long.

- Autistic children have difficulty understanding their listener's perspective, thus creating a lack of insight into the conversation. For example, a person with autism may not understand that someone is using humor or sarcasm. They may interpret the communication word for word and fail to catch the implied meaning.

Repeated behaviors. People with autism might have a fascination with repetitive movement such as spinning wheels, turning on and off lights, or slamming doors.

- Their play may consist of repeatedly spinning tops or watching the same video hundreds of times.
- They may also exhibit stereotyped physical behaviors. These include body rocking, hand flapping, and/or abnormal postures such as toe walking.

Rigid adherence to routines. Autistic children enjoy a set routine. Variations from that routine may upset or frighten them. Even things that appear insignificant, such as taking a different route to school or having a different shape of chocolate chip cookie, will cause them anxiety.

Preoccupation with certain limited topics. Older children and adults are often fascinated by train schedules, weather patterns, dates/calendars, numbers, movie credits, or license plates. For example, they may read books about trains and collect railroad maps and train schedules. They may want to visit rail yards or ride on trains as entertainment. They may discuss trains obsessively.

Preoccupation with parts of objects. Those with autism often seem fascinated by part of an object rather than the whole object itself. This would include such things as the wheels of a car rather than the car itself.

Regression of development. In some children, the first signs of autism may appear during infancy and the

Even things that appear insignificant, such as taking a different route to school or having a different shape of chocolate chip cookie, will cause them anxiety.

disorder is usually diagnosed by the age of 3. In other children, their development appears normal until about 2 years old and then regresses rapidly.

Inconsistent neurologic development. Children with autism develop differently from other children. Typical children develop the full range of neurologic skills (such as language, motor coordination, cognitive ability, and social skills) at about the same rate. Autistic children have an uneven rate of development in these skill areas. Autistic children may have excellent cognitive skills and be able to solve complex math problems and have a wide-ranging vocabulary, but may have difficulty communicating their ideas, taking turns, or reading the emotional content of a person's face or tone of voice.

William's comment:

Our suspicions that Liam may have a problem came in small increments. We noticed when he was about 2 years old that certain noises seemed to bother him, irrespective of the volume level. He grabbed at his ears and cried. At first, we attributed this to a possible ear infection exacerbated by a recent plane trip. The pediatrician was called; he said Liam's ears looked fine, but we should call back in 3 months. A month or two later, a family friend in Los Angeles who works in child care suggested something might be wrong. This friend could not point to anything specific, but mentioned that Liam didn't seem to "pop" the way his peers did. Liam was curious about children his own age or about their toys or snacks, but he didn't engage in reciprocal play. He seemed content to play alone. He did display certain rigidities and, to a slight extent, exhibited a few self-stimulatory behaviors.

15. How do doctors diagnose children with autism?

There is no blood test or X-ray test for diagnosing autism. An accurate diagnosis must be based on observation of the child's communication, behavior, and developmental levels. Autistic children have characteristic behaviors that may be obvious to both parents and clinicians in the first months to years of life. However, because many of the behaviors associated with autism are shared by other disorders, various medical tests may be ordered to rule out or identify other possible causes of the symptoms being exhibited.

To diagnose a child, clinicians must observe a consistent deficit in one of three areas:

1. **Impairment in social functioning**. Clinicians will look for:
   - impairment in many forms of nonverbal expressions (posture, eye contact)
   - failure to develop age-appropriate peer relationships
   - doesn't seek to share enjoyment, interests with others
   - no social or emotional exchange; avoids cuddling or touching

2. **Impairments in communication**. Clinicians will look for:
   - delay or lack of language development
   - inability to begin or sustain a conversation with well-spoken individuals
   - stereotyped/repetitive use of language
   - lack of varied, imaginative play or social actions (age appropriate)

Comprehensive evaluation

A series of tests and observations, formal and informal, conducted for the purpose of determining eligibility for special education and related services and for determining the current level of educational performance.

- lack of response to normal teaching methods or verbal clues
- frequent outbursts and tantrums

3. **Restricted, repetitive patterns of behavior, interest, and activities**. Clinicians will look for:
    - abnormal intensity or focus on a certain stereotyped and restricted behavior
    - inflexible routine of specific nonfunctional ritual
    - stereotyped or repetitive motor mannerisms (flapping arms, spinning their body, walking on their toes)
    - persistent interest with certain parts of objects

Because autism encompasses such a broad spectrum of behaviors, a brief observation in a single setting cannot predict an individual's true abilities. Several evaluations done on different days or in different settings (e.g., home, physician's office, child's school) will yield a more reliable diagnosis. Parental input and developmental history are very important components of making an accurate diagnosis.

Typically, the diagnosis of a child with autism is a two-stage process. The first stage involves developmental screening by a pediatrician during well-child checkups. It is important that the evaluation be performed when the child is feeling well. A sick child may act differently than normal and this makes the observation unreliable.

The second stage entails a **comprehensive evaluation** by a **multidisciplinary team**. The team is composed of a pediatrician, developmental **neurologists**, and speech, physical, and **occupational therapists** as well as a social worker.

Multidisciplinary team

A team whose members come from multiple disciplines; they interact and rely on the others for information and suggestions.

Neurologists

Doctors specializing in medical problems associated with the nervous system, specifically the brain and spinal cord.

Occupational therapists

Individuals who specialize in the analysis of purposeful activity and tasks to minimize the impact of disability on independence in daily living. The therapist then helps the family to better cope with the disorder by adapting the environment and teaching subskills of the missing developmental components.

William's comment:

*A physician, who is a family friend, told me during the time Liam was being evaluated that it didn't take a "rocket scientist" to diagnose autism, but only some experience with the condition and knowledge of the diagnostic criteria. How true that statement was. The developmental pediatrician who spent 10 minutes with my son was able to give me a diagnosis that was consistent with what we got from a child psychologist who spent several hours with him, to a **psychologist** who administered a Bailey test and an ADOS, to another group study at UCLA that administered further tests after even more time spent with him.*

Everything seemed to be consistent, from the 10-minute evaluation to the ones that involved hours and hours of observation.

Psychologist

A specialist in one or more areas of psychology; a field of science that studies the mind and behaviors. Areas of specialty can include psychological testing and practitioners of therapy or counseling.

16. What are screening tools for autism?

Experts point out that it is very important to screen for developmental delays at regular well-child visits. Screening should start when your child is an infant and continue through school age. A common way that pediatricians screen young children is by evaluating their age-appropriate skill development. This refers to skills or milestones that a child is expected to have because most children their age have them. When interviewing the parents of a child suspected of autism, the doctor should ask about loss of speech or a significant decrease in the child's vocabulary or nonverbal communication skills such as pointing or grabbing. The doctor should inquire about any change in social skills, inattentiveness, or an apparent loss of interest in parents or siblings at any age.

When evaluating children for autism, specialists utilize several screening instruments that have been developed to gather information quickly about a child's social and communicative development within medical settings. Some screening tools are based on the examiner's observations of the child. Some evaluations rely solely on parental responses to a questionnaire while others rely on a combination of a parental report and observations.

A screening tool is like a checklist: It lists certain behaviors and abilities of the child and asks the physician to evaluate them. After each evaluation, the physician "scores" that behavior or ability. For example, if "eye contact" were an item on the screening tool, it might be scored like this: 0 = no eye contact, 1 = infrequent, 2 = intermittent, or 3 = full/appropriate eye contact. At the end of the evaluation, the final score is calculated. Certain scores are associated with a diagnosis of autism. Experts validate these screening instruments by using them to evaluate hundreds of children who have been previously diagnosed as autistic and hundreds who are nonautistic children. When the screening instrument can correctly identify the autistic children from the nonautistic children, it is thought to be useful. It is important to note that the results of a screening tool are not sufficient to make a diagnosis of autism. A clinician who is experienced in evaluating children will not make a diagnosis of autism until after completing the following:

1. the parents have been interviewed about the child's medical history, attainment of developmental milestones, and current behavior
2. the child has undergone a thorough physical examination
3. the child has been tested for other diseases that mimic autism

A screening tool only tells the examiner that the child responds in the same way as an autistic child responds.

A screening tool only tells the examiner that the child responds in the same way as an autistic child. It does not tell the examiner why the child responds that way.

It does not tell the examiner why the child responds that way. For example, a child who is hearing impaired may be scored the same as an autistic child. A physician alerted to the results of the screening tool would have to make the appropriate diagnosis after the examination.

17. What are some of the more common autism screening tools that are used today?

The following is a list of the more common screening tools that are used to evaluate children for autism. The screening tools are usually administered by pediatricians, psychologists, or neurologists.

Checklist for Autism in Toddlers (CHAT) This test is a simple screening tool for identification of autistic children at 18 months of age. It has two sections labeled A and B. Section A of the CHAT is a self-administered questionnaire for parents with nine yes-or-no questions addressing the following areas of child development: rough-and-tumble play, social interest, motor development, social play, pretend play, pointing (pointing to ask for something), functional play, and showing (i.e., demonstrating activities or the product of these activities to peers or parents). Section B of the CHAT consists of five items, which are recorded by observation of the children by an experienced clinician. The five items address the child's eye contact, ability to follow a point (gaze monitoring), pretend (pretend play), producing a point (called protodeclarative pointing by experts), and making a tower of blocks.

Modified Checklist for Autism in Toddlers (M-CHAT) The M-CHAT was designed as a simple,

Checklist for Autism in Toddlers (CHAT)

A checklist to be used by general practitioners at 18 months to see if a child has autism.

self-administered, parental questionnaire for use during regular pediatric visits. The more questions a child "fails," the higher his or her risk of having autism. The M-CHAT consists of 23 questions; 9 questions from the original CHAT and an additional 14 questions addressing core symptoms present among young autistic children. The original observational part in CHAT (i.e., section B) is omitted in this screening instrument.

Screening Tool for Autism in Two-Year-Olds (STAT) The STAT is an interactive screening measure for autism. It is designed specifically to differentiate autism from other developmental disorders. The tool is administered through a 20-minute play interaction involving 12 activities. Clinicians using the screening tool sample three areas of interaction with the child, including play (both pretend and reciprocal social play), motor imitation, and nonverbal communicative development.

The Autism Spectrum Screening Questionnaire (ASSQ) The ASSQ is a useful, brief screening device for the identification of ASD in clinical settings. The ASSQ consists of a 27-item checklist that is completed by parents or caretakers of a child who appears to have symptoms characteristic of Asperger syndrome and other high-functioning ASD. It is a valid screening tool for children and adolescents with normal intelligence or mild mental retardation.

Gilliam Autism Rating Scale (GARS) Gilliam Autism Rating Scale (GARS) is a checklist designed to be used by parents, teachers, and professionals to help identify and estimate the severity of symptoms of autism in individuals between the ages of 3 and

Gilliam Autism Rating Scale (GARS)

This is a screening checklist designed to be used by parents, teachers, and professionals to help to identify autistic children.

22 years. It is based on criteria from the American Psychiatric Association and groups items into four sub-tests—**stereotyped behaviors**, communication, social interaction, and an optional test, which describes development in the first 3 years of life.

Childhood Autism Rating Scale (CARS) This screening aids in evaluating a child's body movements, adaptation to change, listening response, verbal communication, and relationship to people. It is suitable for use with children over 2 years of age. The examiner observes the child and obtains relevant information from the parents. The child's behavior is rated on a scale based on deviation from the typical behavior of children of the same age.

Autism Diagnosis Interview–Revised (ADI–R) The ADI–R is a structured interview that contains over 100 items and is conducted with a caregiver. It consists of four main factors: the child's communication, social interaction, repetitive behaviors, and age-of-onset symptoms.

Autism Diagnostic Observation Schedule-Generic (ADOS-G) The ADOS-G is a semistructured, standardized assessment of communication, social interaction, and play or imaginative use of materials for individuals who have been referred because of possible autism or ASD. The ADOS-G is an observational measure used to elicit sociocommunicative behaviors that are often delayed, abnormal, or absent in children with autism. The clinician uses structured activities and materials to provide standard contexts in which social interactions, communication, and other behaviors relevant to ASD can be observed. The ADOS-G can be

Stereotyped behaviors
A common finding with autistic patients. These are repetitive, apparently nonfunctional behaviors, such as rocking and hand flapping; these behaviors are repeated many times.

Childhood Autism Rating Scale (CARS)
An autism screening test developed at Treatment and Education of Autistic and Related Communication-Handicapped Children (TEACCH). The child is rated in 15 areas on a scale up to 4 yielding a total up to 60; ranges are considered to be nonautistic, autistic, and severely autistic.

used to evaluate individuals at different developmental levels and chronological ages.

18. What medical tests should the doctor perform when making a diagnosis of autism?

Customarily, an expert diagnostic team has the responsibility of thoroughly evaluating the child and determining a formal diagnosis. The team will then meet with the parents to explain the results of the evaluation. The clinician may recommend the following tests after a diagnosis of autism has be made:

Formal audiologic evaluation. Various tests such as an **audiogram** and **tympanogram** can indicate whether a child has a hearing impairment. Audiologists (hearing specialists) have methods to test the hearing of any individual by measuring responses such as the turning of the head, blinking, or staring when a sound is presented. Although some hearing loss can cooccur with autism, some children with autism may be incorrectly thought to have such a hearing loss. An additional confounding stiuation occurs when the child has suffered from an ear infection.

Lead screening. This screening is essential for children who remain in the oral-motor stage of development for a long period of time. During this stage, children put anything and everything into their mouths, a behavior called *pica* or *mouthing.* Such children can ingest dangerous amounts of lead even in environments that are usually considered safe. According to several pediatric studies, children with behavioral and/ or developmental problems are more likely to have

Audiogram

The graphic record drawn from the results of hearing tests with an audiometer, which charts the threshold of hearing at various frequencies against sound intensity in decibels.

Tympanogram

The graphic record of a test of the flexibility of the eardrum. It is part of a standard hearing evaluation.

Pica

A perverted or inappropriate appetite for substances not fit as food. These nonfood items include substances that have no nutritional value, such as clay, dried paint chips, starch, or ice.

significantly higher blood-lead concentrations than the general childhood population. Lead, a known—and more importantly, treatable—neurotoxin, would further contribute to the impairment suffered by these children. As a result, experts at many health agencies including the National Center for Environmental Health, the National Institute for Mental Health, the American Academy of Neurology, and the Child Neurology Society recommend routine lead screening for autistic children.

Genetic screening. A screen for fragile X syndrome is appropriate in autistic children. Fragile X syndrome, also known as Martin-Bell syndrome, is a sex-linked genetic abnormality and is the most common form of inherited learning disability and mental retardation. Although not affecting the mother, the genetic defect is carried by her and can be transmitted to her children. It affects approximately 1 in every 1,000 to 2,000 male individuals and the female carrier frequency may be substantially higher. Males afflicted with this syndrome typically have a moderate to severe form of intellectual handicap. Females may also be affected but generally have a mild form of impairment.

Approximately 15 percent to 20 percent of those with fragile X syndrome exhibit autistic-type behaviors, such as poor eye contact, hand flapping or odd gesture movements, hand biting, and poor sensory skills.

Approximately 15 percent to 20 percent of those with fragile X syndrome exhibit autistic-type behaviors, such as poor eye contact, hand flapping or odd gesture movements, hand biting, and poor sensory skills. Behavior problems and speech/language delay are common features of fragile X syndrome. In addition, families are advised to seek genetic counseling to understand the inheritable nature of fragile X syndrome and to discuss with family members the likelihood that other individuals or future offspring may have this disorder.

The diagnosis of Rett syndrome should be considered in females with unexplained moderate to severe mental retardation. If clinically indicated, testing for the MECP2 gene deletion may be obtained. Insufficient evidence exists to recommend testing of females with milder clinical phenotypes or males with moderate or severe developmental delay.

Electroencephalogram or EEG testing. This test should be conducted if a doctor suspects that a child's unusual movements or stereotypic behaviors are the result of a **seizure disorder** or in children whose language and other skills have regressed.

*Brain imaging tests (CT or **MRI** scan).* These tests are rarely helpful toward the diagnosis of autism, but a neurologist might order these tests for some children to rule out other illnesses.

Family functioning evaluation. This evaluation is used to determine the parents' level of understanding of their child's condition in order to offer appropriate counseling and education. A parent educated in the complexities of autism is one of the most important assets an autistic child can have. Most parents' knowledge of autism is rudimentary. After they are told of their child's diagnosis, their reaction is shock, followed by a period of anxiety and depression. This is not the optimal time for parent education. However, the child's physician and other members of the treatment team should help to educate the parents on what they need to know to make the child's and their lives happier and more satisfying. Parents should get recommendations on what further steps they should take for their child. In addition, parents should be provided with the name

Diagnosing Autism

Seizure disorder
Includes any condition of the brain in which there are repeated seizures or convulsions.

MRI (magnetic resonance imaging)
A diagnostic tool that uses radiofrequency waves and a strong magnetic field rather than X-rays to provide remarkably clear and detailed pictures of internal organs and tissues.

Multidisciplinary evaluation team (MET)

A minimum of two persons who are responsible for conducting a comprehensive evaluation of students suspected of being handicapped or children with disabilities being reevaluated.

Sensory integration (SI)

This is a term applied to the way the brain processes sensory stimulation or sensation from the body and then translates that information into specific, planned, coordinated motor activity. Information is received from both internal and external environments through the five senses of vision, touch, taste, hearing, and smell. Our senses are integrated when the nervous system directs this information to the appropriate parts of the brain that enable an individual to attain skills.

or names of professionals who can be contacted if they have further questions. An autistic child can put great stress on a family. Guilt, fear, and depression are common feelings of the parents of newly diagnosed children. It is sometimes helpful to have a professional to help the family recognize and develop coping strategies for these issues.

19. What is a multidisciplinary evaluation team, and how do they help to diagnose an autistic child?

A **multidisciplinary evaluation team (MET)** is a group of certified physicians and therapists from various professional disciplines who specialize in the diagnosis of children with developmental deficits. As has been mentioned, the diagnosis of a child with autism is a two-stage process. The first stage involves developmental screening by a pediatrician during well-child check-ups. The second stage entails a comprehensive evaluation by a multidisciplinary team. The multidisciplinary team typically is composed of one or more representatives of the following specially trained professionals:

Developmental pediatrician. He or she is an expert in the diagnosis and treatment of the health problems of children with developmental delays or handicaps.

Child psychiatrist. This person is a medical doctor who may be involved in the initial diagnosis. In addition, they can prescribe medication and provide help in behavior, emotional adjustment, and social relationships.

Clinical psychologist. A clinical psychologist specializes in understanding the nature and impact of developmental disabilities on a child and family. They may perform psychological and assessment tests and help with behavior modification and social skills training.

Occupational therapist. This specialist focuses on practical, self-help skills that will aid in daily living including dressing and eating. In addition, this therapist may work on **sensory integration (SI)**, coordination of movement, and fine motor skills.

Physical therapist. The **physical therapist (PT)** is an expert in rehabilitation. He or she helps to improve the use of bones, muscles, joints, and nerves to develop the child's muscle strength, coordination, and motor skills.

Speech/language therapist. This professional helps to make diagnoses in speech and swallowing pathology. He or she is focused on the improvement of communication skills including speech and language. The speech therapist also works with children who are unable to speak by utilizing alternate communication strategies such as sign language and picture-aided communication.

Social worker. This person may provide counseling services or act as a case manager by helping to arrange therapeutic services, such as speech, physical, or occupational therapies.

As part of the team's work, a multidisciplinary evaluation might include a complete neurological examination, a comprehensive speech/language/communication evaluation, a cognitive and adaptive behavior evaluation, a sensorimotor and **occupational therapy (OT)** evaluation, and neuropsychological, behavioral, and academic assessments.

Diagnosing Autism

Physical therapist (PT)

A licensed health professional who applies principles, methods, and procedures for analyzing motor or sensorimotor functions to determine the educational significance of the identified areas including areas such as mobility and positioning in order to provide planning, coordination, and the implementation of strategies for eligible individuals.

Occupational therapy (OT)

A type of treatment that assists in the individual's development of fine motor skills that aid in daily living. It also can focus on sensory issues, coordination of movement and balance, and on self-help skills such as dressing, eating with a fork and spoon, grooming, and the like. It can also address issues pertaining to visual perception and hand-eye coordination.

If the parents are suspicious of autism, or not confident in the initial diagnoses made by their pediatrician, they can request an evaluation by this type of multidisciplinary team. If this type of team is not available locally, an excellent alternative for the parents is to have the child evaluated by a pediatrician with a specialty in the evaluation of developmental problems or a pediatric neurologist.

William's comment:

*I've found that not every child requires every one of these services. Although our son receives OT and speech therapy, the area of concentration is primarily behavioral. His **gross motor** skills are for the most part typical; he needs help developing the fine motor skills and his speech at the present time (1 year into services) is starting to expand nicely.*

Gross motor

Movement that involves balance, coordination, and large muscle activity.

20. Are there tests that are not recommended for the diagnosis or management of autism?

The following tests are *not* recommended for the diagnosis or treatment of autism on a routine basis:

Heavy metal testing. Tests for serum levels of mercury, cadmium, or arsenic are not appropriate for the routine evaluation of autism. Although exposure to heavy metals is known to be toxic to humans and may even result in some neurologic disabilities, the cause of autism has not been linked by scientific evidence to exposure to heavy metals. Similarly, tests for such proteins and antibodies as fibrillarin or metallothionein, which may indicate heavy metal exposure, are not appropriate.

Hair analysis. Drug and chemical residues, toxins, and heavy metals in the body embed in hair fiber protein as it grows. Testing hair rather than blood or urine has the advantage of capturing evidence of toxic exposures that may have occurred in recent weeks or months. Hair analysis is used commonly by pathologists and forensic experts to identify such exposures and to identify issues important to occupational health, public health, and the prosecution of crime. The use of hair analysis in the diagnosis of autism is inappropriate for several reasons. These include:

- It presumes that autism is caused by exposures to toxic substances.
- Minute and clinically insignificant amounts of toxic substances may appear in typical and atypical children; finding trace amounts of them in hair does not make a diagnosis.
- The use of hair analysis for ASD diagnosis is not supported by any rigorous scientific study.

Celiac antibodies. Celiac disease (CD) is a lifelong digestive disorder, found in individuals who are genetically susceptible to it. This susceptibility results in damage to the small intestine that ultimately results in interference with the absorption of nutrients. Celiac disease is unique in that a specific food component, gluten, has been identified as the culprit. Gluten is the common name for the offending proteins in specific cereal grains that are harmful to persons with CD. These proteins are found in all forms of wheat (including durum, semolina, spelt, kamut, einkorn, and faro), and related grains: rye, barley, and tritcale. Damage to the mucosal surface of the small intestine is caused by an immune reaction to the ingestion of gluten. Physicians have described the neurological and emotional aspects of patients suffering from celiac disease, which include irritability, anxiety, and withdrawal. Although

Celiac disease (CD)
A disease in which the intestinal lining becomes inflamed after ingestion of foods containing gluten (a protein found in oats, wheat, rye, barley, and triticale). The symptoms in infants and children include diarrhea, slow growth, bloody stools, weight loss, and vomiting. Thought erroneously to be a cause of autism.

there are similarities between these manifestations of celiac disease and autism, the association ends there. Autism is not caused by celiac disease or an allergy to gluten. Testing for antibodies to gluten or intestinal proteins is not appropriate for the diagnosis of autism.

Food allergy testing. A review of Internet sites concentrating on the diagnosis of autism reveals that some practitioners offer an array of tests that supposedly measure antibodies to certain foods or components of foods that these practitioners believe are a cause of autism. These tests may include tests for antibodies to milk proteins, gluten, gliadin, soy proteins, dipeptidylpeptidase IV, and antitransglutaminase. The benefits of this testing are not supported by scientific evidence.

Testing for infectious diseases. Although an infectious agent has long been suspected as a cause of autism, despite exhaustive scientific inquiry, no agent has been identified. Therefore, practitioners who subject children to tests for infectious agents in order to diagnose or treat autism should be viewed with skepticism. Routine testing of children for infectious agents in order to diagnose autism is not recommended. Tests in this category are antibody tests for the following agents: human herpes virus-6, streptococcus M protein, chlamydia species, mycoplasma species, and clostridia neurotoxins as well as yeast and fungal species.

Immune system function testing. Some practitioners recommend tests of immune function for the diagnosis and treatment of autistic children. These tests may include a measure of serum immunoglobulins such as IgG, IgM, IgA, and IgE; the activity and effectiveness of the blood's natural killer cells; and its T4 and T8 lymphocytes or even a measure of a cytokine called tumor necrosis factor. There is no scientific evidence linking the cause of autism to immune function in general or these measures in particular. There is no evidence demonstrating that treating these immunologic mea-sures is an effective therapy for autism.

Vitamin and mineral testing. A deficiency in vitamins and/or minerals has been suggested as the cause of diseases that range from the common cold to cancer. Indeed, there are few diseases whose cause has not been attributed to vitamin deficiency at one time or another. These attributions have rarely, if ever, been supported by scientific evidence. Additionally, while there are a few diseases that are known to result from a vitamin deficiency (e.g., **beriberi**, **pellagra**, **goiter**, and **scurvy**), they are exceedingly rare in Western countries like the United States. Most physicians working in the United States will go through their entire professional lives without seeing an example of a vitamin deficiency disease. In contrast, malnourishment and vitamin deficiency are common in the third world, yet autism is not more frequently diagnosed there. Further, scientific evidence does not support ideas that autism either is caused by vitamin deficiencies or can be cured by supplementing the diet with vitamins and minerals. Vitamin and mineral testing is inappropriate for making the diagnosis of autism or for managing the behavior of children with autism. Tests for vitamin deficiency are not recommended by any accepted medical authorities on autism, nor is there a solid scientific foundation for their use.

William's comment:

Several families we've met at Liam's school report that they've had success with alternative therapies, such as allergy testing and that heavy metal business. When

Beriberi

A specific nutritional deficiency syndrome that occurs from a deficiency of thiamine. It results in painful nerve damage in the hands and feet and heart failure.

Pellagra

A specific nutritional deficiency syndrome that occurs from a deficiency of niacin. It results in gastrointestinal disturbances, skin rashes, and mental disorders. Sometimes called *St. Ignatius Itch* or *alpine scurvy*.

Goiter

A chronic enlargement of the thyroid gland, occurring in areas where food is produced in soil that is low in iodine. Sometimes called *struma*.

Scurvy

A specific nutritional deficiency syndrome characterized by weakness, anemia, swelling of the hands and feet, and ulceration of the gums and loss of the teeth. It is caused by a diet lacking in vitamin C. Also called *scorbutus* and *sea scurvy*.

Vitamin and mineral testing is inappropriate for making the diagnosis of autism or for managing the behavior of children with autism.

I asked them for some published medical studies that support these treatments, they didn't have any. We haven't seen data to substantiate these claims either, though we've looked.

21. Can I wait to have my child tested for autism?

Many parents are reluctant to have their child labeled as autistic. They feel that waiting a few months or a few years will give their child a chance to improve or "get out of this difficult phase." This reluctance is understandable, because autism is a devastating disease and no parent can comfortably embrace this diagnosis. However, putting off an evaluation will not change your child's diagnosis, but it will keep him or her from getting early intervention.

Despite the apprehension that patients and their family may have, once the diagnosis has been made, patients and families often remark how much they have benefited from an official diagnosis of the condition. Getting a definitive diagnosis and in-depth explanation of all the manifestations of the disorder can bring a sense of relief, both for the family—and sometimes for the person themselves—particularly in the case of those at the more able end of the spectrum. A definitive diagnosis also provides the patient, the family, and the school system with the ammunition to argue for the most appropriate services.

Evidence over the last 15 years indicates that intensive early intervention results in improved outcomes in autistic children. This is especially true if the interventions are carried out in optimal educational settings for at least 2 years during the preschool years.

Unfortunately, getting a diagnosis of autism or Asperger syndrome—and most especially an early diagnosis—is often a long and arduous battle. The definitive diagnosis is complicated by parental reluctance and professional unfamiliarity with the condition. However, parents should persevere in this battle for the benefit of their children. Research with children who have, or are at risk for, various disabilities has shown that effective early intervention can substantially reduce their need for specialized services later on. To be effective, however, researchers have found that early intervention must be:

1. comprehensive
2. intensive
3. of long duration
4. individualized
5. delivered directly to children

The principles and methods of applied behavior analysis (ABA) fit these criteria and have produced substantial benefits for many children with autism and pervasive developmental disorder (PDD).

Getting a definitive diagnosis and in-depth explanation of all the manifestations of the disorder can bring a sense of relief, both for the family—and sometimes for the person themself— particularly in the case of those at the more able end of the spectrum.

Diagnosing Autism

PART III

Autism Crisis

What have studies found regarding
vaccinations and autism?

What should a parent do about
childhood immunizations?

Is mercury exposure dangerous?

More . . .

Measles, mumps, and rubella (MMR) vaccine

A vaccine against measles, mumps, and rubella given to children at 18 months and again at around 4 years. Some parents believe it to be directly responsible for autism developing in their child.

22. Has the rate of autism increased since the MMR vaccine has been in use?

Data from a study of California school children have been used to illustrate an increase in cases of autism since the introduction of combined **measles, mumps, and rubella (MMR) vaccine**. However, the data have been presented inaccurately. A scientist reviewing the data lists several reasons why the data are misrepresented. For example:

1. The figures presented are based on absolute numbers of children with autism, not on the rate of autism in the population. Therefore, increases in the population, even if the rate of autism is the same, will result in a higher number of autistic children. Further, since the majority of autism is diagnosed in children, if the number of children in a population increases, even if the total number of the population stays the same, there will be a greater number of autistic children diagnosed. These studies did not account for population growth and changes in the composition of the population when announcing their results.

2. During the period of the study, there were changes in how autism was defined. If the definition of autism were made broader, then more children might meet the criteria for autism. The rate of autism would appear to increase, even if the disabled children were there all along, but had an alternate diagnosis, such as obsessive compulsive disorder or Tourette's syndrome. This study did not control for a changed diagnostic definition of autism, so the results are not reliable.

3. An increased interest in the disease and federal funding for early intervention services occurred dur-

ing this time. Therefore, parents may have been made aware of signs or symptoms of autism and had their children diagnosed earlier. The increased amount of federal funding for early intervention services gave school systems the financial means and social encouragement to have more children evaluated for autism. This may have resulted in children being diagnosed at earlier ages and an increased number of reported cases.

A medical study performed in 2001 used the autism case numbers provided by the California Department of Developmental Services and compared them with early childhood MMR immunization-level estimates for California children. Results showed that for children born from 1980 through 1987, there was no major change in MMR immunization levels with the exception of a small increase in children born in 1988. After this small "bump" in the rate, the immunization rate returned to its previous steady level in children born through 1994. If one assumed that autism was related to immunizations, then one would expect that the rate of autism would reflect the rate of immunizations. However, when the rate of autism in California was compared with the rate of immunization, there was a significant difference. Despite the steady rate of immunization, the number of cases of autism increased markedly, from 44 cases per 100,000 live births in 1980 to 208 cases per 100,000 live births in 1994. Even if one allows that a true increase in autism has occurred and the increase is not due to changes in diagnostic methods, diagnostic categorization, and improved identification of individuals with autism, this analysis shows that receipt of the MMR vaccine is not a factor. This analysis argues against a link between MMR vaccination and autism. Furthermore, there are no proven biological mechanisms that would explain such a relationship. Studies of this kind can never completely rule out rare occurrences of such a reaction.

William's comment:

Our son received all his standard childhood vaccines. We don't feel that had anything to do with his being autistic. We vaccinated our daughter as well, who at this time is 11 months old. We had heard about the possible link between vaccines and autism and worried about it before having our daughter vaccinated. We asked our pediatrician about it and searched the Internet for information on this topic. We ultimately were convinced that it was safe for our daughter, as it was for our son.

23. Do children who get the MMR vaccination have an increased risk for developing autism?

Is there a link between administration of the MMR vaccine and increased risk of autism? No, at least not one that's obvious right now. That's according to an Institute of Medicine report published in May of 2004. The report was authored by a 15-member committee of **epidemiologists**, pediatricians, biostatisticians, and public health experts who convened in Washington, D.C., under the auspices of the Institute of Medicine (IOM).

Epidemiology

The part of medical science that deals with the incidence, distribution, and control of disease in a population.

In recent years, a number of concerns have been raised about the safety of and need for certain immunizations. Although most people realize that vaccines are important for protection against serious infectious diseases, there are some dissenters. According to a study published in 2000 that was based on a national telephone survey, 23% of parents thought that children receive more immunizations than are good for them and 25% thought a child's immune system could be weakened as a result of too many immunizations. This may explain why, even in the United States, where immunization rates are the highest, approximately 1 million pre-school children are not adequately protected against potentially disabling or fatal diseases that can be prevented by immunization.

To address those concerns, the **Centers for Disease Control and Prevention (CDC)** and the National Institutes of Health (NIH) asked the IOM to evaluate the scientific evidence regarding the safety of specific vaccines and whether those vaccines are associated with specific adverse effects.

The IOM reviewed the scientific data available on vaccines and autism up to the year 2004. The scientists in this committee affirmed that vaccines are among the greatest public health accomplishments of the past century. Vaccines have saved millions of lives and prevented millions of people from suffering disabilities. Based on their review, the committee concluded that the body of evidence does *not* support *a causal relationship between the MMR vaccine and autism.* The committee also reviewed the suspected biological mechanisms for vaccine-induced autism and found no evidence to support them.

Even though the committee concedes that it's theoretically possible the vaccine could trigger autism in some toddlers, they say that this phenomenon has not yet been documented and would be extremely rare if it did occur. Therefore, they say that based on their review as well as the overall health benefits of the MMR vaccine, no changes should be made in current federal or state MMR recommendations.

Centers for Disease Control and Prevention (CDC)

A federal agency in the Department of Health and Human Services; located in Atlanta, Georgia; investigates, diagnoses, and tries to control or prevent diseases (especially new and unusual diseases).

Autism Crisis

24. What have studies found regarding the MMR vaccine and autism?

An epidemiologic study is a study of how often a disease occurs in different groups of people and why the disease occurs. Epidemiologic studies do not focus on individuals, but rather look at the frequencies and types of diseases in whole populations of people. These studies are used when trying to learn the reason for increases or deceases in the rates of diseases. In the United States, the CDC is the main source of epidemiologic information. It has conducted many epidemiologic studies of autism and these studies have shown no relationship between MMR vaccination in children and an increased risk of autism. The following is a brief summary of some of the major studies on this topic:

- In 1997, the National Childhood Encephalopathy Study was examined to see if there was any link between measles vaccine and neurological events. The researchers found no indication that measles vaccine contributed to the development of long-term neurological damage, including educational and behavioral deficits (Miller et al., 1997).

Prevalence

The proportion of people with a particular condition or disease within a given population at a given time.

- A study by Gillberg and Heijbel (1998) examined the **prevalence** of autism in children born in Sweden from 1975–1984. There was no difference in the prevalence of autism among children born before the introduction of the MMR vaccine in Sweden and those born after the vaccine was introduced.
- In 1999, the British Committee on Safety of Medicines convened a "Working Party on MMR Vaccine" to conduct a systematic review of reports of autism, gastrointestinal disease, and similar disorders after

receipt of MMR or measles, mumps, **rubella** vaccine. It was concluded that the available information did not support the posited associations between MMR and autism and other disorders.

- Taylor and colleagues (1999) studied 498 children with autism in the United Kingdom and found the age at which they were diagnosed was the same regardless of whether they received the MMR vaccine before or after 18 months of age or whether they were never vaccinated. Importantly, the first signs or diagnoses of autism were not more likely to occur within time periods following MMR vaccination than during other time periods. Also, there was no sudden increase in cases of autism after the introduction of MMR vaccine in the United Kingdom. Such a jump would have been expected if MMR vaccine was causing a substantial increase in autism.

- Kaye and colleagues (2001) assessed the relationship between the risk of autism among children in the United Kingdom and the MMR vaccine. Among a subgroup of boys aged 2–5 years, the risk of autism increased almost fourfold from 1988 to 1993, while MMR vaccination coverage remained constant at approximately 95 percent over these same years.

- Researchers in the United States found that among children born between 1980 and 1994 and enrolled in California kindergartens, there was a 373 percent relative increase in autism cases, though the relative increase in MMR vaccine coverage by the age of 24 months was only 14 percent (Dales et al., 2001).

- Researchers from the United Kingdom conducted a study to test the theory that a new form or new variant of inflammatory bowel disease (IBD) existed. This new variant of IBD had been described as a combination of autism and gastrointestinal

Autism Crisis

symptoms. The neurological and gastrointestinal symptoms seemed to occur shortly after the child received his MMR immunization. Further, the neurological component followed the **developmental regression** type of onset. To study this theory, the researchers gathered medical information on 96 children (95 immunized with MMR) who were born between 1992 and 1995 and who were diagnosed with pervasive developmental disorder. The data from this group of children were compared with data from two other groups of autistic patients. One group of 98 children were born before MMR was ever used, and one group of 68 children were likely to have received MMR vaccine. No evidence was found to support a new syndrome of MMR-induced IBD/autism. For instance, the researchers found that there were no differences between vaccinated and unvaccinated groups with regard to the time when their parents first became concerned about their child's development. Similarly, the rate of developmental regression reported in the vaccinated and unvaccinated groups was not different; therefore, there was no suggestion that developmental regression had increased in frequency since MMR was introduced. Of the 96 children in the first group, no IBD was reported. Furthermore, there was no association found between developmental regression and gastrointestinal symptoms.

- Another group of researchers in the United Kingdom (Taylor et al., 2002) also examined whether the MMR vaccination can be associated with bowel problems and developmental regression in children with autism. The study included 278 cases of children with autism and 195 with atypical autism (cases with many of the features of childhood autism but not

Developmental regression

A form of autism in which infants, after apparently normal development, start to lose language and other skills. This condition is fairly rare and has not been well described nor does it have scientifically established standards for diagnosis.

quite meeting the required criteria for that diagnosis or with atypical features such as onset of symptoms after the age of 3 years). The cases included in this study were born between 1979 and 1998. The proportion of children with developmental regression or bowel symptoms did not change significantly from 1979 to 1988, a period that included the introduction of MMR vaccination in the United Kingdom (1988). No significant difference was found in the rates of bowel problems or developmental regression in children who received the MMR vaccine. There was no difference between the 3 groups in the time to the parent's recognition of developmental delays. The findings of this study do not support the existence of a new type of autism that is caused by the MMR vaccination. Additionally, it suggests that there is no link between autism and MMR vaccinations.

- Madsen and colleagues (2002) conducted a study of all children born in Denmark from January 1991 through December 1998. There were a total of 537,303 children in the study; 440,655 of the children were vaccinated with MMR and 96,648 were not. The researchers did not find a higher risk of autism in the vaccinated than in the unvaccinated groups of children. Furthermore, there was no association between the age at time of vaccination, the amount of time that had passed since vaccination, or the date of vaccination and the development of any autistic disorder. Although there were many more vaccinated than unvaccinated children in the study group, the sample was large enough to contain more statistical power than other MMR and autism studies. Therefore, this study provides strong evidence against the hypothesis that MMR vaccination causes autism.

- DeStefano and associates (2004) conducted a study to see if there was a difference in the age at which children with autism and those without autism received their first MMR vaccination. The study's findings showed that children with autism received their first MMR vaccination at similar ages as children without autism. More information about this study can be found on the CDC's research on vaccines and autism Web page: http://www.cdc.gov/nip/vacsafe/concerns/autism/autism-mmr.htm.

25. What should a parent do about childhood immunizations?

Parents should familiarize themselves first with the information about the importance of vaccinations. For example, we do know that people will become ill and some will die from the diseases vaccines prevent. Measles outbreaks have occurred between 2000 and 2002 in the United Kingdom and Germany following an increase in the number of parents who chose not to have their children vaccinated with the MMR vaccine. Discontinuing a vaccine program based on unproven theories would not be in anyone's best interest.

Parents can become frightened by isolated reports about these vaccines causing long-term health problems.

Parents can become frightened by isolated reports about these vaccines causing long-term health problems. However, careful review reveals that these reports are isolated and not confirmed by scientifically sound research. Detailed medical reviews of health effects reported after receipt of vaccines have often proven to be unrelated to vaccines; rather they have been related to other health factors. Current scientific evidence does not show that MMR vaccine, or any combination of vaccines, causes the development of autism, including regressive forms of autism. Based on this evidence, scientists at the Centers for Disease Control offer some advice to parents:

- **The younger sibling of an autistic child can be vaccinated with MMR or other vaccines safely.** A younger sibling or the child of someone who suffered a vaccine side effect usually can, and should, safely receive the same vaccine. This is especially true because the large majority of side effects after vaccination are local reactions and fever, which do not represent a contraindication.
- **It is not appropriate to delay vaccination of a child until more studies are performed on the autism and vaccinations relationship.** There is no convincing evidence that vaccines such as MMR cause long-term health effects.
- **There does not appear to be any advantage to "splitting" the doses of the MMR vaccines into individual components in order to reduce the risk of autism.** There is no confirmed scientific research or data to indicate that there is any benefit to separating the MMR vaccine into its individual components. The specific issue of the safety of multiple vaccines given as one vaccine was addressed by the Institute of Medicine in 1994 and again in 2002. An IOM Immunization Safety Review Committee concluded that a review of the available scientific evidence does not support the suggestion that the infant immune system is inherently incapable of handling the number of antigens that children are exposed to during routine immunizations. The IOM committee also did not suggest any need to change the current U.S. vaccination schedule for MMR. Pediatricians suggest that splitting the MMR vaccine into three separate doses given at three different times would cause more discomfort from additional

injections and would leave children exposed to potentially serious diseases. For instance, if rubella vaccine were delayed, four million children would be susceptible to rubella for an additional 6 to 12 months. This would potentially allow preventable cases of congenital rubella syndrome (CRS) to occur through transmission of rubella from infected children to pregnant women.

26. Is mercury exposure dangerous?

Yes, exposure to mercury can be dangerous and does result in neurologic illness. Small amounts of mercury are found in the preservative **thimerosal**, which is used in vaccinations. The presence of mercury in vaccinations has led many concerned parents to make a connection between mercury exposure and the development of autism. It may be helpful, therefore, to discuss mercury and its effects on the nervous system in general terms here. In a later section of this book, thimerosal will be discussed at length.

Thimerosal

A compound containing around 50 percent ethylmercury by volume. It is used in vaccines to prevent bacterial and fungal growth.

Mercury occurs naturally in three forms. These are elemental, inorganic, and organic. The elemental form of mercury is the type that used to be found in thermometers; it is silvery, shiny, and looks like liquid metal. The inorganic form comes as mercury bound to another element, such as chlorine or sulfur, in the form of a salt. The last form is organic mercury, such as phenyl-, ethyl-, and methylmercury. Each of these three forms of mercury can cause different levels of illness depending upon the amount of exposure, the route of exposure, and how much is absorbed by the body.

Inorganic mercury enters the body readily, accumulating mostly in the kidney. It enters the central nervous system slowly, but it is also slowly eliminated. Organic mercury compounds are more readily adsorbed and can cross into the brain much more readily than inorganic mercury. The data available from small studies with children have suggested that ethylmercury is less toxic than methylmercury and that it is eliminated from the body more rapidly.

The toxic effects of working with mercury have been well known for millennia. Metal workers and smelters were known to suffer neurologic effects of working with mercury. These effects were also found among hat makers in the 19th century. A mercury solution was commonly used during the process of turning fur into felt, causing the hatters to breathe in the fumes of this highly toxic metal, a situation exacerbated by the poor ventilation of most of the workshops. This led in turn to an accumulation of mercury in the workers' bodies, resulting in symptoms such as drooling, hair loss, uncontrollable muscle trembling and twitching, loss of coordination, a lurching gait, difficulties in forming words, slurred speech, loosening of teeth, memory loss, depression, irritability, and anxiety. In very severe cases, they experienced hallucinations. This became know as the "mad hatter syndrome" in England during the 18th and 19th century, as was popularized in the Mad Hatter character in Lewis Carroll's *Alice in Wonderland*.

During the same period in the United States, Danbury, Connecticut, was known as the "Hat City"; many of its citizens were employed in the hat-making industry. Mercury toxicity was so common in that city that physicians in surrounding areas referred to the neurologic symptoms of confusion, lack of coordination, and trembling hands as "The Danbury Shakes."

One of the most infamous examples of acute mercury exposure in recent history occurred during the 1970s in Iraq. Grain treated with an organic mercury fungicide was the source of contaminated bread. Adults experienced visual disturbances with some subsequent blindness. Prenatal exposures resulted in children with psychomotor retardation manifesting in increased incidence of seizures and delays in learning to walk. During the 1950s in Japan, pregnant women in the Minamata Bay area consumed fish with high levels of methylmercury, resulting in at least 30 cases of infantile cerebral palsy, as well as the deaths of over 100 people.

It should be noted that epidemiologic studies were performed on these populations. Children exposed to high levels of methylmercury while still in their mother's womb experienced significant neurological deficits as well as more subtle developmental delays; however, autism was not observed any more frequently in these populations.

Further, the mercury contained in some vaccines is handled very differently by the body than the methylmercury found in foods such as fish or the mercury from industrial accidents. The ethylmercury in vaccines is eliminated from the body more than two times faster than methylmercury. Therefore, one cannot extrapolate the clinical effects of significant prenatal exposures of methylmercury upon a population of patients with a less intense, postnatal exposure to ethyl-mercury.

27. Does thimerosal cause autism?

Thimerosal has been used as a pharmaceutical preservative since the 1930s and is effective in preventing bacterial and fungal contamination of vaccines. Thimerosal's active ingredient is ethylmercury, which constitutes approximately half of its weight. Before the fall of 1999, there was 25 μg of mercury in each 0.5 mL dose of most diphtheria and tetanus toxoids and acellular pertussis vaccines as well as some *Haemophilus influenzae* type b, influenza, meningococcal, pneumococcal, and rabies vaccines. In addition, there was 12.5 μg of mercury in each dose of the hepatitis B vaccine.

As mentioned in the previous section, data available from studies in children have suggested that ethylmercury is less toxic than methylmercury and that it is eliminated from the body more rapidly.

Although the amount of mercury in each dose of vaccine is very small, the Food and Drug Administration (FDA) determined that under the recommended childhood immunization schedule, infants might be exposed to cumulative doses of mercury that exceed some federal safety guidelines. Additionally, a joint statement issued in July 1999 by the American Academy of Pediatrics and the U.S. Public Health Service recommended the removal of thimerosal from vaccines as soon as possible as a precautionary public health effort to minimize exposure of mercury to infants and children. In 1999, public health officials ordered manufacturers to phase thimerosal out of common vaccines, such as hepatitis and diphtheria, as a precaution. Today thimerosal is all but gone from childhood vaccinations (see Table 1).

In a statement released in May 2004, the IOM Immunization Safety Review Committee reported that, after years of study, they can find no scientific evidence that

Table 1   Thimerosal and Routine Pediatric Vaccines as of the Fall of 2002 Based on FDA Evaluations

Vaccine	Trade Name	Thimerosal Status
DTaP	Infanrix	Free
	Tripedia	Trace* (single dose)
Pneumococcal conjugate	Prevnar	Free
Inactivated poliovirus	IPOL	Free
Varicella (chicken pox)	Varivax	Free
Mumps, measles, and rubella	M-M-R-II	Free
Hepatitis B	Recombivax HB	Free
	Engerix B (GSK)	Trace*
Haemophilus influenzae type b conjugate (Hib)	ActHIB (AP)/OmniHIB	Free
	PedvaxHIB	Free
	HibTITER	Free (single-dose vials)
Hib/Hepatitis B combination	Comvax	Free

*Less than 1 microgram thimerosal per 0.5 mL dose (equivalent to less than 0.5 microgram of mercury per 0.5 mL dose.)

supports an association between autism and thimerosal-containing vaccines, because low doses of thimerosal in human beings are not associated with developmental delay. Additionally, abnormalities in the nervous system that have been associated with exposure to methylmercury have only been shown to occur in prenatal and not postnatal exposure, as occurs in vaccinations. The firm language in this report is indicative of the researchers' confidence and should be compared with earlier IOM reports in 1991, 1994, and 2001, which concluded there was insufficient evidence to accept or reject a link between vaccines and autism.

When considering the risk of small amounts of mercury in vaccinations, one must consider other environmental exposures to mercury that we all have. Mercury occurs naturally in the environment. According to toxicologists at the FDA, approximately 2,700 to 6,000 tons of mercury are released annually into the atmosphere naturally by degassing from the earth's crust and oceans. Another 2,000 to 3,000 tons are released annually into the atmosphere by human activities, primarily from burning household and industrial wastes, and especially from fossil fuels such as coal.

Mercury vapor is easily transported in the atmosphere, deposited on land and water, and then, in part, released again to the atmosphere. Minute amounts of mercury are soluble in bodies of water, where bacteria can cause chemical changes that transform mercury to methylmercury, a more toxic form. Therefore, tiny amounts of mercury exist in the air we breathe, the water we drink, and the food we eat.

PART IV

Autism Therapies and Treatments

How will I know if a new therapy
is right for my child?

Are there therapies besides ABA
that are useful?

More . . .

*Choosing the
right type of
therapy for
your child is
not easy.*

28. How will I know if a new therapy is right for my child?

Choosing the right type of therapy for your child is not easy. Many programs exist whose aim is to improve behavioral symptoms in autistic children. Some even claim to "fix" the underlying problem causing autism.

Unfortunately, not every child responds to even the most effective therapy and some children appear to do well in less-popular treatments. Parents should find out as much about the proposed therapy as possible because not every therapy is based on accepted scientific facts and not every qualified program employs trained teachers and therapists. A parent's investigation should not be limited to exploring the effects of the therapy on the child, but also its affects on the child's parents and siblings.

The Autism Society of America and The National Institute of Mental Health have produced guidelines on what questions a parent should ask about any new therapy. The following are questions based on those guidelines:

Will the treatment result in harm to my child? Have any other children been harmed by this treatment?

How will failure of the treatment affect my child and my family?

Has the treatment been validated scientifically? Can you provide the scientific literature for my review?

How will my child's progress be assessed? Will my child's behavior be closely observed and recorded? Are the assessment procedures specified? Are they scientifically validated?

Are the goals of therapy meaningful to me and/or my child? For example, a therapy whose goal is to decrease self-stimulatory behavior by 10 percent may not be worth participating in.

How will the treatment be integrated into my child's current program? Does it have a holistic approach, acknowledging that the child has other interests and goals? A parent should not become so infatuated with a given treatment that functional curriculum, vocational life, and social skills are ignored.

How successful has the program been for other children?

How many children have gone on to placement in a regular school and how have they performed?

What are the qualifications of the staff members? How many of them will be working with my child? Do staff members have training and experience in working with children and adolescents with autism?

How are activities planned and organized? Who plans them?

Are there predictable daily schedules and routines?

How much individual attention will my child receive?

Will my child be given tasks and rewards that are personally motivating? What will the rewards be? Can that reward system be duplicated in the home? Will the program prepare me to continue the therapy at home?

Is the therapeutic environment designed to minimize distractions?

What is the financial cost and time commitment of this therapy?

Where will the therapy take place? Does that location require a license or certification to perform this therapy?

A professional and reputable therapist or therapeutic program should answer these questions easily and openly. A failure to answer to your satisfaction should give you pause and prompt further investigation before allowing your child to undergo this treatment.

William's comment:

Our son is in an intense ABA program. We have found that the quality and intensity of the ABA therapy vary across the nonpublic agencies that provide care for autistic children.

29. What is applied behavioral analysis?

Behavioral interventions are those actions, processes, or programs designed to change the behavior of children with autism. The theory underpinning most behavioral interventions can be explained simply as behaviors that are rewarded tend to be repeated more frequently than behaviors that are ignored or punished.

Using a system of trials and rewards to change behavior in a particular setting or for a particular task is called *behavioral conditioning* or *behavioral modification*. Behavioral modification programs have been developed and employed in the treatment of autistic children. The most popular and arguably the most effective program is called applied behavioral analysis (ABA).

Ivar Lovaas, a doctor of psychology from UCLA, first developed this program and is referred to as "the father of ABA." Dr. Lovaas understood the importance of creating a process of positive reinforcement for the development of desired behaviors. He further theorized that every interaction that an autistic child has is an opportunity to either reinforce good behaviors or ignore them, leading to less-acceptable behaviors. He felt that the current school or institutional environment provided therapies that were neither intense enough nor long enough. He needed to develop a program that intensified the number and duration of these behavioral interactions. With these realizations, Dr. Lovaas formulated a comprehensive therapeutic and educational plan that has grown into ABA.

ABA is the design, implementation, and evaluation of environmental modifications to produce socially significant improvements in behavior. ABA includes the use of direct observation, measurement, and functional analysis of the relations between environment and behavior. During this therapy, the therapist gives the child a task to perform. Every task given to the child consists of a request to perform a specific action, a response from the child, and a reaction from the therapist. Tasks are broken down into short simple pieces or trials. When a task has been successfully completed, a reward is offered, reinforcing the behavior or task. It is not just about correcting behaviors but is designed to teach skills, from basic ones such as washing and dressing to more involved ones such as social interaction. A recent study has shown that up to half of children who underwent full-time intensive discrete trial therapy had behavioral improvement.

Applied behavior analysis has become a well-developed discipline in its own right. It has a mature body of knowledge, established standards for practice, distinct methods of service, recognized experience, and educational requirements for practice. As far back as 1981,

Applied behavior analysis has become a well-developed discipline in its own right.

85

Special education

Specially designed instruction, at no cost to the parents, to meet the unique educational needs of the student with disabilities and to develop the maximum potential of that student.

ABA was identified as the treatment of choice for autistic behavior and is commonly taught to **special education** teachers who work with autistic kids.

William's comment:

Our son attends a program in southern California. The founders of the program were involved in the Young Autism Project study conducted by Ivar Lovaas. After interviewing many programs in our area, we feel that the people who run Liam's program are the New York Yankees in a field of Triple A players. We are very fortunate to have gotten our son in there. It's not just that the program offers some ABA therapy, but I feel it is also crucial that a child gets qualified and interested providers who can give him the necessary number of hours (Lovaas suggests 40).

A parent should, after researching the best programs in their area, get on the list for services and then call every few days for as long as it takes. Be persistent. The old adage of "the squeaky wheel" seemed to apply to my wife's nonstop inquiries.

30. What is sensory integration therapy?

Sensory integration (SI) therapy is a sensory-motor treatment for children with autism. Dr. A. Jean Ayres developed this therapy based on her understanding of neurologic development and autism. Dr. Ayers recognized that children with autism frequently had sensory difficulties. These difficulties included being either over- or underresponsive to sensory stimuli or lacking the ability to integrate the senses. She noted that children with autism may be startled by a slight sound (hypersensitivity) or may totally tune out external stimuli, such as language (underresponsive). Dr. Ayers postulated that self-stimulation and stereotypic activities that are characteristic of many autistic children are related to this sensory dysfunction. She further theorized that the brain has the ability to change or improve its functioning (a property called *neural plasticity*) and that improvement in brain functioning could be achieved through a therapy directed at appropriately integrating the sensory stimuli. SI therapy, she felt, could result in a reduction in the rates of self-stimulation and self-injurious behaviors.

SI therapy, usually administered by occupational, physical, or speech therapists, focuses on desensitizing the child and helping them reorganize sensory information. It is obvious then that before proceeding with any sensory integration therapy, it is important that the therapist observe the child and have a clear understanding of the child's sensitivities.

SI activities include swinging in a hammock, spinning in circles on a chair, applying brushes to various parts of the body, and engaging in balance activities. These activities are hypothesized to correct the underlying neurological deficits producing the perceptual-motor problems witnessed in many individuals with autism. In other words, SI therapy is not designed to teach the child new physical or motor activities, but to correct fundamental sensory-motor dysfunctions underlying the disorder in order to increase the individual's capacity for learning new activities.

Critics of Dr. Ayers' SI therapy state that her therapy is based on an unproven theory of the cause of autism and an unproven theory of treatment. These critics state that the results of current research do not support sensory integration as an effective treatment for children with autism, developmental delays, or mental retardation. Further, according to the limited research to date, there is no proof that SI therapy is responsible for any positive change in an autistic child's behaviors or skills. In fact, in at least one study, SI therapy was shown to increase self-injurious behaviors.

William's comment:

We have been told the same. When services are given, it makes no sense to offer both ABA and SI, as SI therapy takes time away from the more effective ABA therapy.

31. What is TEACCH?

Treatment and Education of Autistic and Related Communication-Handicapped Children (TEACCH)

A structured educational program that targets both the strengths and weaknesses that are often seen in children with autism. It is a project of the University of North Carolina.

TEACCH is an acronym for **T**reatment and **E**ducation of **A**utistic and Related **C**ommunication-Handicapped **CH**ildren. It was developed at the School of Medicine at the University of North Carolina in the 1970s and was the first comprehensive state-wide community-based program of services for children and adults with autism and other similar developmental disorders.

Today, TEACCH provides a wide range of services to a broad spectrum of toddlers, children, adolescents, adults, and their families including diagnosis and assessment, individualized treatment programs, special education, social skills training, vocational training, school consultations, parent training and counseling, and the facilitation of parent group activities. TEACCH offers a structured teaching approach based on the idea that the environment should be adapted to the child with autism, not the child to the environment. The program is based upon a thorough understanding of the child's functioning level. Teaching strategies are designed to accommodate a child's identified strengths and weaknesses. TEACCH does not employ a single therapeutic method for a child's treatment; rather, it uses the best available approaches and methods for an education with the goal of having that child achieve their maximum level of autonomy. Special emphasis is placed on helping people with autism and their families live together more effectively by reducing or removing "autistic behaviors." Some of the unique aspects of this program include:

- **Improved adaptation**. They employ two strategies of adaptation. They work to improve a child's skills by means of education, and they modify the child's environment. These strategies accommodate the child's deficits and decrease his or her stressors.
- **Parent collaboration**. Parents are considered as co-therapists for children in this program. TEACCH therapists work with parents to teach them therapeutic techniques and advise them about how to modify the home environment for the benefit of their child, so that techniques utilized in school can be continued at home.
- **Assessment for individualized treatment**. Through regular assessment of the child's abilities, unique educational programs are designed.
- **Structured teaching**. TEACCH programs use a structured teaching environment. Research demonstrated that children with autism benefit more from a structured educational environment than from free approaches.

The TEACCH approach is not without its critics. Some feel that the program is too structured. Others complain that autistic children are often distracted by the charts, organizational aids, and schedules the program utilizes. Finally, critics assert that TEACCH discourages **mainstreaming** of autistic children.

Mainstreaming
The concept that students with disabilities should be integrated with their nondisabled peers to the maximum extent possible, when appropriate to the needs of the child with a disability. Mainstreaming is one point on a continuum of educational options. The term is sometimes used synonymously with *inclusion*.

32. I've heard of an educational model called Floor Time. What is it?

Child psychiatrist

A physician (medical doctor) specializing in mental, emotional, or behavior disorders in children and adolescents; is qualified to prescribe medications.

Floor Time is an educational model developed by **child psychiatrist** Stanley Greenspan. It is sometimes referred to as Developmental Individual-Difference, Relationship-Based Model. DIR/Floor Time utilizes interactive experiences, which are directed by the autistic child, as a therapeutic activity. Floor Time therapy is conducted in a low-stimulus environment with the duration of these interactive experiences ranging from 2 to 5 hours a day.

DIR/Floor Time is related to the concept of play therapy, wherein the child's activity of interest (play) is employed to develop other positive social skills. By following the child's lead, the therapist or parent builds on what the child does to encourage more interactions. Greenspan's Floor Time educational model is thought to build an increasingly larger number and intensity of interaction between a child and an adult. This child-therapist interaction progresses in a developmentally based sequence and is thought to result in the autistic child's emotional development. Greenspan has described six stages of emotional development (or milestones) that children meet to develop a foundation for more advanced learning. According to Greenspan, these milestones are:

1. The dual ability to take an interest in the sights, sounds, and sensations of the world and to calm oneself down.

2. The ability to engage in relationships with other people.

3. The ability to engage in two-way communication with gestures.

4. The ability to create complex gestures and to string together a series of actions into an elaborate and deliberate problem-solving experience.

5. The ability to create ideas.

6. The ability to build bridges between ideas to make them reality-based and logical.

Greenspan theorized that by using Floor Time, parents and educators can help the child move up through these developmental milestones. Floor Time is focused on the emotional development of the autistic child rather than the cognitive development. It does not specifically address areas such as speech development or motor development, as traditional therapies do. Floor Time is frequently used for a child's daily playtime in conjunction with other methods such as ABA.

It is important to note that the outcomes of children treated with Greenspan's Floor Time educational model have not been subjected to adequate scientific scrutiny. Therefore, no statement can be made about the effectiveness of this therapy.

William's comment:

Again, same thing. Dr. Quinn is dead on in our opinion. We've had experiences with a speech therapist who advocated Floor Time. We feel that a good ABA therapist will have more success in getting a child to speak than a licensed speech pathologist.

33. What is facilitated communication?

Facilitated communication is a technique that purports to allow people with autism who have severe language deficits to express themselves at near-normal and

Facilitated communication

A discredited therapeutic method that employs a person (the facilitator) and an assistive communication device to help autistic children to communicate and eventually overcome autistic behaviors. This theory lacks scientific support. Also known as *facilitated communication training*.

normal levels. It is based on the idea that the person is unable to communicate because of a movement disorder, not because of a lack of communication skills. An Australian patient's aid, named Rosemary Crossley, developed this system in the 1970s while trying to help a patient with cerebral palsy communicate.

The technique involves a facilitator who places his or her hand over that of the patient's hand, arm, or wrist, which is placed on a board or keyboard with letters, words, or pictures. The facilitator provides only backward resistance to the disabled person's hand. Using this technique, the patient is allegedly able to communicate through his or her hand to the hand of the facilitator, which then is guided to a letter, word, or picture, spelling out words or expressing complete thoughts.

Proponents of facilitated communication claim that with this technique, verbal and nonverbal individuals with autism can communicate at levels previously thought to be impossible. They insist that although physical assistance is necessary during the typing process, the facilitator does not influence the selection of letters.

Facilitated communication has been used with both children and adults with autism in a variety of contexts. It has been used during the administration of intelligence tests, and individuals who previously performed in the severe and profound range of mental retardation have been reclassified as having normal intelligence. Based on the quality of facilitated output, children with autism and severe mental retardation are being placed in regular classrooms and are reported to be performing academic tasks at grade level.

One can imagine the emotional effects on parents who previously thought their child was profoundly retarded or brain damaged and are now told that their child has a lively intellect and a rich "life of the mind." Through their facilitators, previously mute patients recite poems, carry on high-level intellectual conversations, or simply communicate. Parents are grateful to discover that their child is not hopelessly retarded but is either normal or above normal in intelligence. Facilitated communication allows their children to demonstrate their intelligence; it provides them with a vehicle previously denied them. Facilitated communication may seem a godsend to desperate or forlorn parents.

Facilitated communication may seem a godsend to desperate or forlorn parents.

Critics ask an important question: "Is it really their child who is communicating or is it the ideas or thoughts of the facilitator that are being communicated?" Critics point out that, to date, no empirical database has proven that facilitated communication is that of the individual and not that of the facilitator. Facilitated communication has not been scientifically validated by any objective scientific group, and most skeptics believe that the only one doing the communication is the facilitator.

Indeed, it is a highly controversial technique with many opponents. Organizations such as the American Association of Mental Retardation and the American Academy of Child & Adolescent Psychiatry and the American Psychological Association have adopted formal positions opposing the acceptance of facilitated communication. Accumulated peer-reviewed, empirically based research studies have not supported the effectiveness of facilitated communication.

34. What is the Picture Exchange Communication System?

One of the commonest disabilities found in autistic children is an impaired ability to communicate. While some children with autism will develop verbal language, others may never talk. A program that either helped develop language abilities or that provided an alternate means of communication was needed. To satisfy these needs, the augmented communication program called the **Picture Exchange Communication System (PECS)** was developed.

The PECS system originated at the Delaware Autistic Program. It was specifically developed for use with young nonverbal children or children with limited functional speech who have autism or other social communication challenges.

PECS uses ABA-based methods to teach children to exchange a picture for something they want such as an item or an activity. People using PECS are taught to approach and give a picture of a desired item to a communicative partner in exchange for that item. Children progress through sequenced phases, enabling them to communicate within a social context. While advancing through the phases of PECS, the student learns to sequence words to create sentences. Pointing to pictures is discouraged as pointing does not require interaction with a person. Using PECS, students learn to gain the attention of the communication partner in order to make a request. Because the student learns to spontaneously initiate communicative exchanges, PECS is used with children or adults who are not yet initiating requests or offering comments.

Picture Exchange Communication System (PECS)

A system created to aid the communication of nonverbal autistic patients. PECS employs a simple picture card system used to encourage autistic people to communicate their needs.

The advantage to PECS is that it is clear, intentional, and initiated by the child. The child hands you a picture and his or her request is immediately understood. It also makes it easy for the child with autism to communicate with anyone. A further advantage is that a PECS program does not require a lengthy prerequisite training period or expensive materials. It can be taught to parents and other therapists for use in all the child's environments.

35. Are there other therapies that are useful in the treatment of behavioral symptoms in autistic children?

Yes, there are other therapies that *may* be helpful in the treatment of autism symptoms. As is mentioned in other sections of this book, there is no cure for autism nor is there a standard therapy that works for all or even most people with autism. Keep in mind, however, as with most complementary approaches, there is little scientific research that supports the efficacy of these therapies.

A number of different treatment approaches have evolved over time as we have learned more about autism. Though early educational intervention is recognized as a key to improving the lives of individuals with autism, some parents and professionals believe that other treatment approaches may be helpful also. These complementary approaches can play an important role in improving communications skills and reducing behavioral symptoms associated with autism. These complementary therapies may include different forms of exercise, music, art, or animal therapy and may be done on an individual basis or integrated into an educational program.

All these therapies utilize a child's interest and focus on a particular activity or topic to teach other skills such as socialization and communication. They can also help by providing the child with a sense of enjoyment, accomplishment, and cooperation that extends outside of the therapy sessions. These therapies are a nonthreatening way for a child with autism to develop a positive relationship with a therapist in a safe environment.

As with any therapy or treatment approach, it is important to gather information about the treatment and make an informed decision. Parents should make sure that the program is designed and run by a therapist familiar with autistic children and that there are clear goals for the therapeutic sessions, outside of learning a particular artistic, musical, or athletic skill.

Exercise and athletic therapy. Autistic children, like their typical counterparts, have both the interest and energy for athletics. To the extent that the child is interested and derives pleasure from the physical activity, that activity can be used to increase physical and emotional well-being as well as serving as a forum for teaching skills, such as the social aspects of playing in groups and communication. Athletic programs can include activities such as swimming, running, playing softball and basketball, or even practicing yoga.

William's comment:

Liam's greatest deficits at this time appear to be social. Ideally, directing him into sports will provide us with more opportunities for social moments/interactions. We have a tee ball set-up and encourage him to "take a few cuts." He'll hit the ball, then run to the base, after which he will get a lot of positive reinforcement from his mother and me. We

As with any therapy or treatment approach, it is important to gather information about the treatment and make an informed decision.

have a little basketball set-up as well. Our goal is that when he's old enough, we'll try to have him join an organized athletic team.

As for sports serving as OT, with Liam we're a little more concerned with the finer motor skills, as opposed to gross. But it definitely doesn't hurt.

Art and music therapy. The use of art and music are particularly helpful in improving sensory integration because they can provide tactile, visual, and auditory stimulation in a controlled environment. Art therapy can be used to encourage hand–eye coordination through drawing and painting. It can increase tactile stimulation when the children use modeling clay, plaster, and wax. The development of their own artwork and the interpretation of the artwork of others provide the autistic child with a nonverbal, symbolic method of self-expression. Listening to music and hearing and singing songs are helpful in developing speech and language comprehension. Learning to play an instrument helps the child to enhance the length of concentration and increase focus on a productive activity.

William's comment:

Part of Liam's therapy includes learning how to do little art projects. He also does a weekly music class, but this is more for his enjoyment, as he loves music.

Animal therapy. Animals can provide an intense stimulus to children. The animals can focus a child's attention and enhance their ability to listen and learn. Animal therapy may include training dogs, playing with hamsters, horseback riding, or swimming with dolphins. Physical benefits from these types of therapies include aerobic exercise from running, riding, or swimming as well as improved motor coordination and muscle development. Intellectually, experimental studies have shown that animal therapy is associated with enhanced learning and retention of information when compared to the class setting. Psychologically, children are more receptive to socialization such as turn taking and are more interested and willing to communicate if it means getting an extra ride or time with an animal they're interested in. Children may also enjoy these therapy sessions and develop feelings of accomplishment, well-being, and self-confidence from them.

Many of these programs make unfounded claims about their benefits to autistic people. It should be clear that these therapies do not treat autism per se. They do not raise a child's IQ, improve anti-social behavior, or decrease self-stimulatory behaviors.

PART V

Medication and the Treatment of Autism

Are medications useful in treating the behavioral problems of autistic children?

What types of medications are used to treat autistic children?

How are anxiety and depression treated in an autistic person?

More . . .

36. Are medications useful in treating the behavioral problems of autistic children?

No medication can cure autism. Some autistic children may require medication for a short time and others require life-long treatment to help with their behavior or other symptoms. Most autistic children require no medication at all. Many distressing symptoms and unusual behaviors can be improved without the medication. Reducing these distressing symptoms enhances the individual's ability to participate in educational and community programs, as well as reducing the stress experienced by the parents or caregivers.

Behavioral problems in autistic children can range from hyperactivity, motor and vocal tics, difficulty with transitioning from task to task, uncooperativeness, or defiance to aggression, uncontrollable tantrums, and self-abusive behavior, such as biting of the hands and arms. Although most behavioral problems are amenable to behavior modification techniques such as ABA, refractory, severe, or dangerous behaviors may require medication to treat them effectively.

When a child develops new behaviors—especially when the onset is abrupt or the behavior is violent, parents and caregivers should be vigilant for identifiable causes of the behavior, such as conflicts at school with teachers, therapists, or classmates; allergies; physical ailments or injuries; or more serious illnesses. Even behavioral changes that occur slowly, that are sometimes dismissed as "typical autistic behavior," can be caused by a reparable problem in the environment. Because communication is a problem with autistic children and adults, they may find it difficult to tell their caregivers

No medication can cure autism.

that they are feeling sick or are in pain. This frustration may manifest itself as aggression or self-injury, especially if the person is pressured to continue with daily routine or work activities.

When a child exhibits a deterioration of behavior, although it may eventually be attributed to their underlying autism, parents should consider the following causes first:

- *Social conflict*: Consult with teachers and therapists to see if there have been issues in your child's school environment.
- *Infections*: Physical ailments such as earaches, tooth abscesses, and influenza may be causing problems.
- *Unrecognized injury*: Hyperactive children are prone to minor injuries and sometimes more serious injuries. An inability to communicate or explain the injury can result in unrecognized injuries going unnoticed by parents.

Dr. Quinn's comment:

Our child suffered a serious fracture of his upper arm that went unrecognized for 2 days, and whose only symptom was emotional withdrawal and decreased interest in his favorite meals.

- *Medication side effects*: Many common medications, such as cold or allergy medication, can cause behavioral changes in autistic children. Paradoxically, medications used to improve behavior can sometimes worsen it.
- *Worsening of a chronic medical condition*: Behavior changes may indicate a worsening of a chronic medical condition such migraine headache, stomach ulcers, hemorrhoids, rheumatoid arthritis, or Crohn's disease.

Discussing new behaviors, as well as any other symptoms (such as fever, diarrhea, lethargy, or change in gait), with the child's pediatrician is important. Every effort must be made in these cases to treat the underlying condition medically before treating the behaviors unnecessarily with sedatives, antidepressants, or tranquilizers.

37. What types of medications are used to treat autistic children?

The types of medications used to treat an autistic child depend on the symptoms as well as any other condition that may contribute to unacceptable behavior. Medications commonly prescribed to treat the behaviors of autistic children include antidepressants, anticonvulsants, **neuroleptic** medications (also known as antipsychotic medications), sedatives, and stimulants.

Neuroleptic

A class of drug that includes Haldol and Risperdal. Also called *antipsychotic medication*.

These medications all can have serious side effects and are not prescribed lightly by concerned physicians. Although most medications can be used safely for long periods of time without harm, the use of any medication is associated with health risks. Parents should be aware of the risks to the child as well as the likely benefit to the child. Treating a child with medication should only be undertaken after the parents (and the child, when appropriate) have balanced the risks and benefits of the medication. Parents need to be made aware of all the possible side effects of any new medication as they will be observing the child most closely and can aid the treating physician in decisions about adjusting the dose of medication or eliminating it.

38. Is there anything I should do before giving my child a medication?

Behavioral problems, such as aggression, self-injurious behavior, and severe tantrums, can keep the person with autism from functioning effectively at home or in school. Physicians can use medications to treat these behavioral problems. When your child is treated with medication, you should observe the following rules:

1. *Consult experienced physicians.* A child with autism may not respond in the same way to medications as typically developing children. Given the complexity of medications, drug interactions, and the unpredictability of how each patient may react to a particular drug, parents should seek out and work with a physician who has experience in treating autistic children with these medications. This physician should be able to tell the parents what the appropriate dosage for their child is and how it should be administered (e.g., pills, liquid, or injection).

2. *Observe closely.* Like any person taking a new medication, an autistic child should be monitored closely by the parents and medical professionals. You should ask the physician how your child will be monitored and by whom. Ask your physician about what signs or symptoms you should look for that may signal a problem or what laboratory tests are required before starting the drug and during treatment.

3. *Begin with low doses.* Because the amount and severity of medication side effects tend to heighten with an increase in the dose of the medication, doctors should prescribe the lowest dose possible that is effective. The doctor may begin with a low dose and then observe its effects on your child's behavior

for weeks or months. The doctor may have to make several adjustments to get the right dose that optimizes behavior and minimizes side effects.

4. *Be aware of the side effects of the medications prescribed.* When medication is being discussed or prescribed, ask about the safety of its use in children with autism. Ask the doctor about any side effects the medication may have and if there are any long-term consequences to the use of the medication. It is helpful to keep a record of how your child responds to the medication at what dose. The product insert that comes with your child's medication lists the drug's indications, side effects, and monitoring requirements; parents should read this and discuss any concerns they have with the doctor. Some people keep the product inserts in a small notebook to be used as a reference. This is especially useful when your child is prescribed several medications.

5. *Be aware of drug or food interactions.* The physician should be made aware of any other medications your child is taking, including over-the-counter cold medications, home remedies, or nutritional supplements. Ask the physician if there are there possible interactions with other drugs, vitamins, or foods.

Antipsychotic medications have been used to treat severe behavioral problems in autistic children.

39. Are antipsychotic medications helpful in the treatment of autism?

Antipsychotic medications have been used to treat severe behavioral problems in autistic children. These medications work by reducing the activity in the brain of the neurotransmitter dopamine. The use of antipsychotic medication in autism is not intended to imply that autism and psychosis are in any way related. However, these medications, used to treat psychotic behaviors in psychiatric patients, also have been shown to be effective with autism. Antipsychotic medications are divided into two classes: typical and atypical.

Typical antipsychotic medications. Some examples of the typical antipsychotics include **haloperidol** (Haldol), thioridazine, fluphenazine, and chlorpromazine. The most commonly used medication in this group is haloperidol.

- *Haloperidol* was found in more than one study to be more effective than a placebo in treating serious behavioral problems in autistic patients.

Haloperidol
A medication that has been found to decrease symptoms of agitation, hyper-activity, aggression, stereotyped behav-ior, and affective lability.

Unlike some prescription drugs that must be taken several times during the day, some antipsychotic medications can be taken just once a day. In order to reduce daytime side effects such as sleepiness, some medications can be taken at bedtime. Some antipsychotic medications are available in "depot" forms that can be injected once or twice a month. A "depot form" of an injectable drug is formulated by the manufacturers to be released slowly from the injection site into the bloodstream. This prolongs the effect of a single injection, allowing a larger dose to be administered less frequently.

Most side effects of antipsychotic medications are mild; many common ones lessen or disappear after the first few weeks of treatment. These include drowsiness, rapid heartbeat, and dizziness when changing position. Infrequent side effects can include muscle stiffness and abnormal muscle tics and facial movements called *tardive dyskinesia.* Tardive dyskinesia is a condition associated with the use of antipsychotic medication. It is characterized by involuntary, rhythmic movements of the face, jaw, mouth, and tongue, such as lip pursing, chewing movements, or protrusion of the tongue. These facial movements are sometimes accompanied by involuntary jerky or writhing motions of the trunk, arms, and legs.

Atypical antipsychotic medication. The early typical antipsychotic medications often had unpleasant side effects, such as muscle stiffness, tremor, and abnormal movements. Looking for a way to avoid these side effects, researchers continued their search for better drugs. This research resulted in the development of the **atypical antipsychotic medications**. The atypical antipsychotic medications are generally more effective in treating behavioral symptoms, but are not without their own side effects, which include dizziness, rapid heartbeat, and fainting. Atypicals are also known for their propensity to induce weight gain. Some examples of aytpical antipsychotics include **Risperdal** (risperidone), Seroquel (quetiapine), Zyprexa (olanzapine), Zeldox (ziprasidone), Clozaril (clozapine), and Abilify (aripiprazole). The medication most frequently studied in children is risperidone.

- *Risperidone* has a wealth of data supporting its efficacy in the improvement of behavioral disturbances in autistic children. It helps to lessen aggression, agitation, and explosive behaviors. In the systematic review on the use of atypical antipsychotics in autism, researchers concluded that risperidone might be effective in reducing hyperactivity, aggression, and repetitive behaviors, often without inducing severe adverse reactions. The most common side effects were increased appetite, weight gain, and sedation.

- *Olanzapine* (Zyprexa) and *ziprasidone* (Geodon) have been studied in autistic children with encouraging results. The most important adverse events reported with olanzapine were weight gain, loss of strength (asthenia), and increased appetite. Ziprasidone has not been associated with significant weight gain.

40. I've heard that antiseizure medications can be helpful in treating some behavior problems associated with autism. Is that true?

Yes. Antiseizure medications (also called *anticonvulsants*) are another group of medications that have demonstrated effectiveness in treating behavioral symptoms in autistic patients.

Although anticonvulsants are prescribed mainly for epilepsy, the mood-stabilizing and behavioral effects of this class of medication are increasingly being studied. Researchers have noticed that while treating autistic children for their seizures, their aggressive behaviors improved while on the antiseizure medication. How these medications work to curb aggressive behavior is unknown. Although these medications are designed to treat seizure activity, physicians will often prescribe them for children who suffer from both a seizure disorder as well as **behavioral disorders**. These medications have numerous side effects, some of which are severe. These include problems with liver function as well as with production of blood in the bone marrow. Therefore, each of these medications requires regular blood

Behavioral disorders

Disorders affecting behavior and emotional well-being.

testing in order to ensure that liver or bone marrow damage does not occur.

Antiseizure medications commonly prescribed for autistic children include:

- *Depakote* (divalproex sodium). In addition to treating seizures, Depakote is indicated in the treatment of bipolar disorder (manic-depression) as well as migraine headaches. It has the benefits of lessening explosive behaviors and aggression in patients with autism. Common side effects include sedation and upset stomach. Unusual, but dangerous, side effects include liver failure, pancreatitis, and low platelet counts. Frequent blood tests must be done to monitor the blood count, liver, and pancreatic enzymes. Signs of irregularities should prompt a discontinuation of the medication and consultation with the prescribing physician.
- *Tegretol* (carbamazapine). Like Depakote, Tegretol is indicated for treatment of seizures and bipolar disorder. Some studies demonstrate improvement in behavioral symptoms in autistic children. Side effects are numerous and include drowsiness, headache, dizziness, fatigue, and allergic skin reactions. A rare side effect is to decrease the bone marrow's ability to produce blood cells. As with Depakote, regular visits to the doctor are necessary for blood tests.
- *Neurontin* (Gabapentin) and *lamictal* (Lamotrigine) are other medications that show potential but have not been studied sufficiently to be recommended for use with children. They appear to provide the same benefits as Depakote, as well as the same side effects, but insufficient data exist on their overall effect.

41. How are anxiety and depression treated in an autistic person?

Although depression has been described in autistic children, limited information is available about how frequently depression occurs. Experts believe that the rate of depression in autistic children is higher than in typical children. Common types of treatment for depression include the **selective serotonin reuptake inhibitors (SSRIs)** and the tricyclic antidepressants.

The SSRIs are the medications most often prescribed for symptoms of anxiety, depression, and/or obsessive-compulsive disorder (OCD). These medications are generally considered safe and have few side effects. Treatment with these medications is associated with decreased frequency of repetitive, ritualistic behavior and improvement in aggression and self-injurious behaviors. Use of SSRIs has been reported to improve a child's eye contact and social interactions. The FDA is studying and analyzing data to understand how to use the SSRIs safely, effectively, and at the lowest dose possible. Some examples of the SSRIs include:

- *Fluoxetine* (Prozac). A selective **serotonin** reuptake inhibitor (SSRI) type of antidepressant; it has been approved by the FDA for both OCD and depression in children ages 7 and older.
- *Fluvoxamine* (Luvox). A selective serotonin reuptake inhibitor (SSRI) type of antidepressant; it has been approved by the FDA for both OCD and depression in children ages 8 and older. Although not as popular as fluoxetine, fluvoxamine has a sedating effect that is not found in Prozac. This may prove to be an advantage in hyperactive children.

Selective serotonin reuptake inhibitor (SSRI)

A class of drugs used as antidepressants. Functionally, they increase the levels of serotonin in the body. These drugs can be dangerous if mixed with other drugs such as other antidepressants, illicit drugs, some antihistamines, antibiotics, and calcium-channel blockers. Some examples of SSRIs are Prozac, Zoloft, and Paxil.

Serotonin

A neurotransmitter implicated in the behavioral-physiological processes of sleep, pain and sensory perception, motor function, appetite, learning, and memory.

Convulsions

Involuntary spasms especially those affecting the full body.

• *Sertraline* (Zoloft). A selective serotonin reuptake inhibitor (SSRI) type of antidepressant; it has been approved by the FDA for both OCD and depression in children ages 6 and older. It causes less agitation than Prozac but is associated with weight gain.

Tricyclic antidepressants, while effective, are associated with many more side effects and are not as safe to use as the SSRIs. Tricyclic agents should be used with extreme caution in patients with a history of **convulsions** or epilepsy. These agents are known to increase the tendency for seizures. Tricyclics should also be used with caution in children with irregular heartbeats, because they can cause a worsening of irregular heartbeats (cardiac arrhythmias). A frequently used medication in this class is clomipramine.

• *Clomipramine* (Anafranil). Clomipramine is a tricyclic antidepressant agent with both antidepressant and antiobsessional properties. Like other tricyclic antidepressant agents, clomipramine inhibits norepinephrine and serotonin uptake into central nerve terminals. It is approved for treatment of depression and obsessive compulsive disorder in children ages 10 and older. Clomipramine also appears to have a mild sedative effect that may be helpful in alleviating the anxiety component often accompanying depression.

Other drugs, such as Elavil (amitriptyline hydrochloride) and Wellbutrin (buproprion hydrochloride), have not been studied as much as others but may have a role in treating depression as well as the behavioral symptoms in autism. Keep in mind that all these drugs have potential side effects, which should be discussed with the treating physician before treatment is started. Parents should be alerted to these side effects so that they are able to discuss the effects of the medication with the physician, who may adjust the dose or stop the medication.

42. What medications are used to treat seizures in autistic children?

Seizure disorder, a condition also known as epilepsy, occurs more commonly in autistic children than in typically developed children. In fact, one in four persons with autism has a seizure disorder. The onset of seizure activity in the autistic usually occurs during infancy, childhood, or adolescence.

Seizures result from an abnormal electrical discharge in the brain. Causes of this abnormal electrical activity can include an imbalance of the salt or sugar in the blood, head injuries, infections of the brain and its coverings, or, rarely, brain tumors. Often the cause of the seizure is unknown. Epilepsy is the diagnosis given to patients who suffer from repeated seizures that occur without an identifiable cause.

Seizures in autistic patients are commonly of two varieties. The majority of seizures in autistic children are of the *grand mal* type, while a smaller number suffer from *petite mal* seizures.

Grand mal seizures (also known as *tonic-clonic seizures or convulsions*). A grand mal seizure is a common type of seizure. Patients suffering from a seizure can be recognized by the symptoms that may include a loss of consciousness and loss of motor control that, if they are standing, may make them fall down. They frequently lose control of their bowel or bladder and will soil their clothes after a seizure. However, the most characteristic sign of a seizure disorder is rhythmic convulsions of the whole body. These seizures rarely last more than a minute or two. After the seizure, the patient is often confused and lethargic and may complain of headache.

Petite mal seizures (also known as *absence seizure*). Unlike a grand mal seizure, an absence seizure causes a loss of consciousness that is usually 30 seconds or less and is barely noticeable. Rather than falling down, the person simply stops moving or speaking, stares straight ahead blankly, and does not respond to questions. During a petit mal seizure, small jerks sometimes occur involving the facial muscles, jaw, or hands. Each seizure lasts only seconds or minutes, but hundreds may occur each day and the patient may be unaware that a seizure has occurred. A person who experiences a petit mal seizure can usually resume normal activities immediately after the seizure ends.

Parents concerned about symptoms that may be seizure related should have their child evaluated by a pediatric neurologist, who may recommend a test that measures brain waves. This test is called an electroencephalogram or EEG.

The treatment of seizures in autistic patients varies depending on their needs and the severity of the condition. When medication is indicated, the treatment of seizure disorder requires one or more anticonvulsants. Although anticonvulsants usually reduce the number of seizures, they cannot always eliminate them. Anticonvulsants commonly prescribed include carbamazepine (Tegretol), lamotrigine (Lamictal), topiramate (Topamax), and valproic acid (Depakote).

As noted in the previous section, these medications are associated with many side effects; therefore, frequent monitoring of medication levels in the blood as well as blood cell counts and liver and pancreatic enzyme levels are required.

43. What are some treatments for involuntary movements, vocalizations, and Tourette's syndrome associated with autism?

Tourette's syndrome is an inherited neurological disorder that is characterized by involuntary movements and vocalizations. Involuntary movements or vocalizations also occur more commonly in autistic children when compared with the general population. Autism and Tourette's may be linked by a common biochemical derangement and can occur together in some children. Medications are currently the only effective treatments for these conditions. These medications include:

High blood pressure medications: Researchers have found low doses of clonidine or guanfacine to be useful in treating autistic people with these types of movement disorders. As a consequence, clonidine hydrochloride (Catapres) and guanfacine (Tenex), two alpha 2-adrenergic agonists, are the most frequently prescribed medications for tics in the United States. Clonidine was developed as a blood pressure medication, but was found to decrease the rate and severity of tics. Though originally indicated for persons with high blood pressure, clonidine and guanfacine can generally be taken by individuals with normal blood pressure. Clonidine is available in tablet and sustained-release (transdermal) patch form. Like all medications, clonidine does have some side effects that can be problematic. The most

Tourette's syndrome is an inherited neurological disorder that is characterized by involuntary movements and vocalizations.

problematic side effects reported have been dry mouth and drowsiness or somnolence. Guanfacine has the same side effect profile, although the drowsiness tends to be somewhat less. Although many patients adjust to the medication's side effects, others don't and discontinue the medication. Even if clonidine does work, it may take time before its effect builds up in the system.

Antidepressant drugs: Preliminary results from a small study of five autistic children show a significant improvement in movement disorders using the antidepressant drug clomipramine. (It is sold under the brand name Anafranil in the United States.) Anafranil, a chemical cousin of tricyclic antidepressant medications such as Tofranil and Elavil, is commonly used to treat people who suffer from obsessions and compulsions.

Antipsychotic drugs: Medications such as olanzapine (Zyprexa) and risperidone (Risperdal) can help reduce tics and other symptoms of Tourette's syndrome. Nevertheless, they often produce unpleasant side effects, such as drooling, muscular rigidity, tremor, and lack of facial expression. Drugs used to treat Parkinson's disease often can reduce these side effects. Prescription of low doses of antipsychotic medications may be necessary for resistant cases.

PART VI

Alternative Treatments for Autism

Is there any harm in trying unproven
treatments on my child?

Are dietary interventions helpful
to autistic children?

More . . .

44. Is there any harm in trying unproven treatments on my child?

The ideal treatment for an autistic child would have the following characteristics:

- Curative (rather than just improving symptoms)
- Effective in all children (not just some a certain type or degree of autism)
- Quick (it would not take years of therapy to accomplish)
- Easy to administer (a pill or an injection)
- Risk free (no side effects)
- Inexpensive (cost would be minimal or free)

Currently, no treatment for autism can achieve this ideal. Even the most promising treatments for autism often fall far short. Additionally, years of intensive treatment with an unexplored therapy could leave the autistic individual with substantial additional impairments. Despite this, parents desperate to help their autistic child can be lured into trying unproven treatments. It is natural for parents, educators, and even mental health professionals to ask: "What harm is there in trying this new treatment?" Unfortunately, the answer to this question is "great harm." There are good reasons to be cautious; some of the more common reasons are listed here:

Expense: No treatment is without cost, even if a practitioner were not to charge for the unproven treatment. Costs a parent can incur while trying an unproven treatment include:

- *Direct financial cost*: Unproven treatments are often quite expensive. Money spent on an unproven treatment takes money away from more effective treatments or from other financial obligations of the parent. When employing unproven therapy, the time to a "cure" or "substantial improvement" is unknown. Without this information, there is a tendency for parents to continue therapy long past the point where an honest professional would suggest that the therapy is not working. The hope for a cure keeps many parents spending money long after a reasonable chance of success has passed. Adding financial stress to a household with an autistic child is unwise.

- *Opportunity costs*: The time and resources parents spend on an unproven therapy are time and resources that could have been spent on an intervention with a greater likelihood of success. For example, many experts feel that early intervention programs that use accepted behavioral modification techniques, such as applied behavioral analysis, are particularly effective. However, if the child spends the early years in an unproven and ultimately ineffective therapy, then the opportunity for early intervention is lost.

- *Psychological costs*: Parents who seek "cures" or dramatic improvements in their children from unproven therapies are often disappointed. A repeated experience with treatments that are promoted with much fanfare but turn out to be ineffective can cause family members of autistic individuals to become depressed or unnecessarily cynical about new treatments, even those that are legitimate interventions.

Physical harm: Physical harm can come from pharmacological, dietary, and behavioral interventions. The annals of the FDA are filled with numerous examples of substances that were initially believed to be useful and without harmful side effects that turned out to be

Alternative Treatments for Autism

quite harmful. Examples range from the birth defects associated with the fertility drug thalidomide to heart valve damage associated with the use of the diet drugs fenfluramine and dexfenfluramine (i.e., Fen Fen). Some practitioners are now recommending the use of substances like **secretin** and dimethylglycine (DMG) for the treatment of autism. The effects of long-term use have not been investigated and are unknown.

Dietary interventions that recommend a very limited diet (such as a gluten-free diet) are difficult to achieve and may deprive children of needed nutrients. Other diets that encourage high-dose vitamin or mineral supplementation have sometimes led to sickness or death.

Even behavioral interventions are not without risk of harm. In the past, some behavioral interventions have encouraged parents to use physical punishment to decrease the amount of socially inappropriate behavior. In some cases, this punishment has resulted in allegations of child abuse by family members. Overly restrictive or intense behavioral interventions can increase a child's frustration level and result in an increase in autistic behaviors, with further regression from socially acceptable behaviors.

Dr. Quinn's comment:

I am not suggesting that parents and professionals not be allowed to explore a range of treatment options. What is suggested is that they do so with as much information as possible, and armed with an attitude of healthy skepticism. For several reasons, such skepticism is particularly important in considering treatments for autism as it acts as a balance to the strong desire to do "something" for your child.

Secretin

A polypeptide neurotransmitter (chemical messenger); one of the hormones that controls digestion, increasing the volume and bicarbonate content of secreted pancreatic juices.

Finally and perhaps most importantly, one must always be aware of the potential for harm.

William's comment:

There is no mountain a parent won't climb barefoot if they think it would be beneficial to their autistic child. It takes real discipline to plot out a course of action and to stick to it. Financial liabilities, as Dr. Quinn mentions, can be tremendous in proven therapies (ABA). It's not a great idea to go looking for something new and unproven.

45. Are dietary interventions helpful to autistic children?

Yes, but, not in the way some parents think. Autistic children can suffer problems from a poor diet. On the one hand, they can be very picky eaters, limiting their diet to only a few food items that may not contain all the nutrients a child needs. A balanced and nutritious diet is important and should be a goal for parents. On the other hand, obesity can become a problem for some autistic children. As they get older and are able to open the refrigerator and reach pantry cabinets, it can become difficult to put limits on how much they eat. Further, encouraging children to exercise safely is a challenge for most parents. Discussions with the child's pediatrician or a licensed dietician can be helpful in designing an appropriate diet for an autistic child.

However, this is often not the dietary advice some parents seek. In an effort to do everything possible to help their children, many parents continually seek new diets as a form of treatment for symptoms or as a cure for autism. Unfortunately, there is no scientific evidence

Autistic children can suffer problems from a poor diet.

that supports any diet as a treatment for behavioral symptoms or a cure for autism.

Not all advertised treatments are concocted by charlatans with the intent to defraud desperate parents. Some treatments are developed by reputable therapists or by parents of a child with autism who sincerely believe their diet will help. It may even have appeared to help in some child treated with it. An unproven treatment may help one child, yet may lack any benefit to another or may even be harmful. Without subjecting each diet to scientific scrutiny, no statement can be made about the treatment's effectiveness or safety.

Scientific scrutiny implies that an experimental trial is performed on a large group of autistic children by objective researchers. Typically, researchers randomly assign the autistic children into two equal groups of children of similar ages and disabilities. One group would receive an intervention, such as a new diet, medication, or nutritional supplement. The other group would receive a sham treatment or placebo pill. None of the examining doctors, the parents, or the autistic children would know who was getting the real treatment. After the trial was over and all the children were evaluated, the doctors would learn which group received the "active treatment" and which group received the placebo or sham treatment. If there were no detectable differences between the groups, then the treatment would be determined to be ineffective. If there were a significant improvement in the treatment group, it would imply that the treatment was effective in improving autistic symptoms. This type of experiment is called a *randomized, double-blind trial* and it is the basis for all new treatments accepted by the FDA. Unfortunately, most dietary treatments have not been subjected to this type of evaluation.

46. What are some common dietary interventions used to treat autism?

Most dietary interventions used to treat autism are based on one of two unproven assumptions. The first is that food allergies cause the symptoms of autism and the second is that autism is caused by a deficiency of a specific vitamin or mineral.

Food allergies. An idea that has gained currency among some parents holds that autism is caused by an allergy to gluten or casein. Gluten is an insoluble protein that is found in the seeds of various cereal plants—wheat, oats, rye, and barley. Gluten is a mixture of various proteins including gliadin, glutenin, and prolamins. Casein is the principal protein in milk and chief constituent in cheese. Because cereals and milk are found in many of the foods we eat, following a **gluten-free, casein-free diet** is difficult. No scientific evidence supports the idea that a low or gluten-free diet improves the symptoms of autism. There is a similar lack of evidence for casein-free diets.

Dietary supplements. Some parents feel that supplementing their child's diet with vitamins and minerals, such as vitamin B_6 and magnesium, is beneficial for an autistic child. The results of research studies on these supplements are mixed; some children respond positively, some negatively, some not at all or very little. Most authorities on autism do not recommend this.

William's comment:

I have heard about this type of therapy—where a kid is cured of his autism by changing his diet. Of the people who have told me of these cures, none knew the parents or child who was cured personally. I have to question if they were autistic to begin with. I'll believe it when I see it.

Gluten-free/ casein-free diet

A diet believed by some to help improve the symptoms of autism. It involves elimination of gluten (a protein found in wheat and other grains) and casein (a protein found in milk) from the diet. It is believed, although not proven, that the undigested portion of these proteins acts like a chemical in the brain, producing symptoms in children with autism. No scientific evidence supports this theory.

Control of dietary yeast. Some have hypothesized that children suffer from autism because of an overgrowth of yeast in their intestinal tract or bloodstream. They believe that this overgrowth may contribute to or cause the behavioral and medical problems in individuals with autism, such as confusion, hyperactivity, stomach problems, and fatigue. The use of nutritional supplements, antifungal drugs, and/or a yeast-free diet has been suggested as a way to reduce the behavioral problems. No scientific data support this theory of disease or treatment and it is not recommended.

It must be stressed again that the cause of autism is unknown and that dietary interventions have not been shown to improve the symptoms of children with autism.

If, despite what is written here, parents decide to implement a special diet or to give their child a dietary supplement, they should be sure that the child's nutritional status is measured carefully. Discussing the proposed diet with a physician or qualified dietitian is recommended.

47. Is secretin helpful in treating the symptoms of autism?

Secretin is a hormone produced by the small intestines that helps in digestion. It is currently approved by the FDA as a single injection to aid in diagnosis of a gastrointestinal problem. Some parents have reported that after undergoing a diagnostic test that utilized secretin, their child's symptoms improved. Some physicians have reported that after injections of secretin, a patient has shown improvement in autism symptoms, including sleep patterns, eye contact, language skills, and alertness.

Eager parents have sought out practitioners to administer secretin to their children. Equally eager, but less scrupulous physicians have offered injections and infusions of secretin. These treatments were often given in complex regimens, over long periods of time, and often at great cost to the parents in terms of finances, time, convenience, and emotion. The child was subjected to the discomfort of injections and the fear of the unknown as well as being taken away from traditionally and scientifically valid treatments. Ultimately, little change was noted in the child and the parents were emotionally crushed.

The scientific basis of how secretin might work has not been described. Despite this, the theory that it can affect improvement in behaviors has been subjected to multiple scientific tests. Disappointingly, the several studies funded by the National Institute of Child Health and Human Development (NICHD) have found no statistically significant improvements in autistic symptoms when compared to patients who received a placebo.

It is also important to remember that secretin is approved by the FDA for a single dose; there are no data on the safety of repeated doses over time.

48. Is naltrexone helpful in treating autism?

In the late 1970s, studies of neonatal animals exposed to high levels of opiates revealed that they exhibited autistic-like withdrawal after they were born. Further, opiate-treated animals exhibited unusual hyperactivity and repetitious (perseverative) behaviors much like autistic children. Additionally, researchers have noted similar behavior patterns between autistics and opiate

Researchers have noted similar behavior patterns between autistics and opiate addicts such as social withdrawal, self-stimulation, and high levels of pain tolerance.

addicts such as social withdrawal, self-stimulation, and high levels of pain tolerance.

Scientists are aware that the body produces its own natural opiates, called **endorphins**. *Endorphins* are produced in the body to decrease pain and can be experienced after hard exercise; for example, in the so-called "runner's high." Some researchers theorized that autistic individuals have too much beta-endorphin in their central nervous system and that the self-stimulatory and self-injurious behavior of typical autistic children is an attempt to increase the production of those endogenous opiates (or endorphins.) This is referred to as the **addiction theory of autism**.

The use of the opiate antagonist, **naltrexone**, to treat autism followed. This addiction theory goes on to suggest that naltrexone, a drug that blocks the effects of both external and internally produced opiates, should have a beneficial effect on autistic children. Using naltrexone in the treatment of autism appeared reasonable because it is known to antagonize opiate receptor activity in the brain and is an FDA-approved treatment for substance-use disorders such as heroin addiction and alcoholism as well as opiate overdoses.

Although primarily a safe drug, naltrexone is not without side effects. When studied in alcoholic populations and in healthy volunteers in clinical pharmacology studies, results have suggested that a small fraction of patients may experience an opioid withdrawal-like symptom complex consisting of tearfulness; mild nausea; abdominal cramps; restlessness; anxiety; and bone, joint, and muscle pain; as well as nasal congestion symptoms. The safety of long-term use of naltrexone in autistic people has not been studied.

Endorphins

Implicated in the regulation of pain perception, social and emotional behaviors, and motor activity. Once thought to be a cause of autism.

Addiction theory of autism

The belief that an overabundance of naturally produced opioid compounds (called endorphins or encephalins) is the cause of autism.

Naltrexone

This drug blocks brain cell receptors for opioids, natural opium-like substances produced by the body that may be abnormally high in autism.

A large number of uncontrolled reports support the effectiveness of naltrexone in the treatment of autism. However, the five controlled trials that are available are far less encouraging.

The value of naltrexone treatment as a routine trial for hyperactive, self-injurious autistic children remains debatable. Despite encouraging anecdotal reports describing behavioral improvement in one or a few patients, when subjected to strict scientific studies, the results were less impressive. At present, eight double-blind placebo-controlled trials exist on this topic. They conclude that naltrexone is at best minimally effective in the treatment of autism. Naltrexone should not be utilized as a first-line drug in the treatment of autism and generally is not employed by specialists in autism.

49. What is chelation therapy?

Heavy metal toxicity can cause a wide range of problems including severe injury to the body organs and the brain. **Chelation** therapy is used to treat these toxic exposures. Chelation therapy involves the use of chemical compounds to bind several types of heavy metals that are present in toxic concentrations in the body. These medications can be injected into the vein, the muscle, or can be taken by mouth. They work by binding to the toxic compound and then are easily excreted from the body in the urine or feces. Chelation therapy was first developed by the U.S. Navy as a way of removing toxic metals from the bodies of military personnel exposed to high concentrations of lead during the 1940s. Since that time, it has been used in the treatment of people exposed to lead paint particles and other environmental exposures. Chelating agents are approved for use by the

Chelation

The formation of a complex between a metal ion and two or more polar groupings of a single molecule. For example in heme, the Fe^{2+} ion is chelated by the porphyrin ring. Chelation can be used to remove an ion from participation in **biological** reactions, as in the chelation of Ca^{2+} of blood by EDTA, which thus acts as an anticoagulant. A chelating agent will bind with metals in order to try to release them from the body.

Alternative Treatments for Autism

FDA, but have limited medical indications. Chelation therapy is medically indicated when a patient is exposed to toxic levels of heavy metals such as iron, arsenic, lead, and mercury. It is a recommended treatment by the American Academy of Family Practice and the American Academy of Pediatrics for this purpose. The conditions that chelation therapy is used to treat include:

- *Lead toxicity* most commonly occurs with young children exposed to old houses with lead paint dust or chips. Occupational exposure (soldering, welders, smelters, battery reclamation) is also a risk. Lead screening for children has now become a standard part of a doctor's visit for children in most states.
- *Mercury toxicity* almost always occurs with high-risk occupational exposures including dental workers, manufacturers of batteries and thermometers, tannery work/taxidermy, and contaminated seafood.
- *Arsenic poisoning* usually occurs from exposure to insecticides, herbicides, rodent poisons, veterinary parasitic medications, or intentional poisoning.
- *Iron toxicity* usually occurs when a child ingests an overdose of iron pills. Iron pills are used as a supplement to dietary iron in treatment of patients with low blood counts (anemia).

Although there are other heavy metals (cadmium, manganese, aluminum, cobalt, zinc, nickel, copper, and magnesium) that can cause illness when a patient is exposed to high doses, these exposures are extremely rare.

Common chelating agents include:

- **Desfuroxamine mesylate**: used for iron toxicity; intravenous is the preferred route of administration

- **Dimercaprol (BAL)**: the preferred agent for treating arsenic and mercury toxicity, given as an intramuscular injection
- **DMSA**: an analogue of dimercaprol that can be given orally for lead and arsenic poisoning
- **D-penicillamine**: an oral chelating agent used for lead, arsenic, or mercury poisoning; much less expensive but not as effective as DMSA
- **Calcium disodium versante (CaNa$_2$-EDTA)**: can be used in conjunction with BAL in lead toxicity; never used alone in treating lead toxicity because it chelates only extracellular, not intracellular, lead
- **Succimer**: an orally active, heavy metal–chelating agent; indicated for the treatment of lead poisoning in pediatric patients

Diagnosis of heavy metal toxicity is serious and must be made by a physician based on clinical symptoms in conjunction with laboratory testing. Chelating agents can be toxic, causing rashes and liver and kidney injury as well as bone marrow suppression with low white blood cell counts (neutropenia). While these agents have no effect on diseases such as atherosclerosis, Alzheimer's disease, Parkinson's disease, or autism, they can remove other essential metals from the blood such as iron, zinc, copper, and magnesium. Deficiencies resulting from chelation agents can cause adverse health effects. Therefore, chelating agents should not be used unless heavy metal toxicity has been diagnosed in a reputable laboratory and therapy is monitored by a qualified physician.

50. Can chelation therapy help my autistic child?

Concerns about mercury contained in vaccinations have prompted concerned parents and others to theorize that mercury is the cause of autism. As a result, some practitioners have begun using chelating agents as a treatment for autism. According to this theory, once the mercury is removed, its toxic effects are eliminated, and the individual begins to show improvement in autistic symptoms.

The most vocal proponent of chelation therapy for diseases other than heavy metal toxicity is the American College for Advancement in Medicine (ACAM). In contrast, the overwhelming opinion of the traditional medical community is that effectiveness of chelating agents used to treat other diseases is unproven and should be avoided. The traditional medical community does not recognize ACAM as an authoritative source of clinical information.

The few studies that exist attempt to demonstrate the effectiveness of chelating agents in the treatment of cardiovascular disease. There are no studies that demonstrate the effectiveness of chelating agents in improving autistic symptoms or other symptoms of developmental diseases. The Autism Biomedical Information Network lists chelation as an unproven treatment. They point out that no reliable research studies have been made on many treatments being offered as alternatives to traditional autism treatments, and that most of the information available on their effectiveness is anecdotal rather than based on valid scientific research techniques. Cure Autism Now (CAN), a leading autism research organization, called for research proposals to investigate the effectiveness of chelation therapy in autism treatment. They state that since no research studies exist that validate the claims of those who support chelation as a treatment of autism, chelation should be considered unproven and its safety and effectiveness still undetermined.

Compounding the lack of supporting scientific evidence is the mercenary behavior of practitioners using chelating agents. A typical therapeutic program is long and costly. Treatment costs can run between $75 and $125 per session. Parents are told that their child must undergo between 20 and 100 treatments before showing results. Because this is an unapproved treatment and not covered by health insurance, parents are expected to pay in cash. Other physicians point out that some chelation therapists attempt to secure insurance coverage by misrepresenting the patient's treatment to the insurance companies, therefore practicing insurance fraud rather than medicine.

Until valid research is conducted and chelation is approved for use in the treatment of autism, it is recommended that it be avoided.

Treatment costs can run between $75 and $125 per session.

PART VII

State and Federal Entitlement Programs

What is SSI?

How does the government decide
if a child is disabled?

What health care services are
available to my child?

More . . .

51. How long does it take for Social Security to determine if my child is disabled?

The disability evaluation process generally takes several months. However, the law includes special provisions for people (including children) signing up for **supplemental security income (SSI)** disability whose condition is so severe that they are presumed to be disabled. In these cases, SSI benefits are paid for up to 6 months while the formal disability decision is being made. Keep in mind, these payments can be made only if the child meets the other eligibility factors.

Supplemental security income (SSI)

A federal assistance program administered by the Social Security Administration for aged, blind, and disabled persons under Title XVI of the Social Security Act to guarantee a certain level of income. SSI recipients have contributed nothing or not enough to the Social Security System to be able to receive benefits on their own earnings record.

The following are some diagnoses where the government will make a presumption of disability and will make immediate SSI payments:

- HIV infection
- Total blindness
- Total deafness (in some cases)
- Cerebral palsy (in some cases)
- Down syndrome
- Muscular dystrophy (in some cases)
- Mental retardation
- Diabetes (with amputation of one foot)
- Amputation of two limbs
- Amputation of leg at the hip

If parents take these payments and the government later decides that the child's disability is not severe enough to qualify for SSI, the benefits do *not* have to be paid back.

52. What is SSI?

Supplemental security income (SSI) is a need-based program that provides cash assistance to people with limited income and assets who are age 65 or older, disabled, or blind. Children can qualify if they meet Social Security's definition of disability. SSI is funded by the federal government and is administered by the Social Security Administration (SSA).

As its name implies, SSI *supplements* a person's income up to a certain level. The level varies from one state to another and can go up every year based on cost-of-living increases. Recipients of this benefit also receive **Medicaid**. Your local Social Security office can tell you more about the SSI benefit levels in your state.

Supplemental security income is not Social Security. Social Security is a program that provides retirement benefits, survivors' benefits, and disability benefits to people who have worked enough to qualify or to their spouses and children. The benefits are based in part on payments made to Social Security while working. Most people over the age of 65 receive Social Security payments.

Medicaid

Title XIX of the federal Social Security Act and 42 CFR 430 to 456; pays for medical care for low-income persons; is a state-administered program.

53. How does the government decide if a child is disabled?

While your local Social Security office decides if your child's income and assets are within the SSI limits, all documents and evidence pertaining to the disability are sent to a state office, usually called the Disability Determination Service (DDS). There, a team consisting of a disability evaluation specialist and a medical or psychological consultant reviews your child's case to decide if he or she meets the definition of disability.

In these cases, SSI benefits are paid for up to 6 months while the formal disability decision is being made.

If the available records are not thorough enough for the DDS team to make a decision, you may be asked to take your child to a special examination that Social

Security will pay for. It is very important that you do this and that your child puts forth his or her best effort during the examination.

As you can see, it is imperative to collect, organize, and safely store all of your child's school records as well as records of psychological, neurological, and medical examinations. They will continue to be examined as long as your child requires medical care or insurance benefits.

The law states that a child will be considered disabled if he or she has a physical or mental condition (or a combination of conditions) that results in "marked and severe functional limitations." The condition must last or be expected to last at least 12 months or be expected to result in the child's death. In addition, the child must not be working at a job that is considered to be substantial work by the government.

To make this decision, the disability evaluation specialist first checks to see if a child's disability can be found in a special listing of impairments that is contained in Social Security's regulations. These listings are descriptions of symptoms, signs, or laboratory findings of more than 100 physical and mental problems, such as cerebral palsy, mental retardation, or muscular dystrophy, that are severe enough to disable a child. The child's condition does not have to be one of the conditions on the list. But if the symptoms, signs, or laboratory findings of the child's condition are the same as, or medically equal in severity to, the listing, your child is considered disabled for SSI purposes. If your child's impairment(s) does not meet or medically equal a listing, the DDS then decides whether it "functionally equals" the listings. They assess the effects of the condition or combination of conditions on your child's ability to perform daily activities by comparing your child's functioning to that of children the same age who do not have impairments. To do this, they consider questions such as:

- What activities is your child able to perform?
- Which activities are limited in comparison with those of same-age peers?
- What type and amount of help does your child need to complete age-appropriate activities?

To determine whether your child's impairment causes "marked and severe functional limitations," the disability evaluation team obtains evidence from a wide variety of sources who have knowledge of your child's condition and how it affects his or her ability to function on a day-to-day basis and over time. These sources include, but are not limited to, the doctors and other health professionals who treat your child, teachers, counselors, therapists, and social workers. A finding of disability will not be based solely on your statements or on the fact that your child is, or is not, enrolled in special education classes.

54. What are the eligibility criteria for Supplemental Security Income (SSI)?

SSI benefits are payable to disabled children under age 18 who have limited income and resources or who come from homes with limited income and resources.

This means that:

- the child must meet the government's definition of being financially needy, or he or she must live in a home where the parents have limited income and assets.

- A child may be eligible for SSI benefits based on disability from the date of birth; there is no minimum age requirement.
- A child may be eligible for SSI benefits based on disability until attainment of age 18.
- At age 18, the government evaluates a person's impairments against its definition of disability for adults.

When evaluating a disabled child under 18 years of age for SSI eligibility, the government looks at the parent's income and assets. If the parents' assets and income fall below a predetermined level and the child has a condition that meets the government's definition of disability, then the child is eligible for SSI benefits. This applies to children who live at home or who are away at school but return home occasionally and are subject to parental control. This process is called *deeming* of income and assets.

If a child was ineligible for SSI benefits because of parental income, his eligibility status can change when he reaches 18 years of age. A child who was not eligible for SSI before his or her 18th birthday because the parents' income or assets exceeded the government's criteria, may become eligible at age 18. The federal government does not consider the parents' income and assets when deciding if a child over 18 is eligible for SSI.

For the autistic child who receives SSI benefits, turning 18 may have little effect on those benefits. Ordinarily, a child's SSI benefits end when a child reaches age 18 (or 19 if the child is a full-time student). However, for the child who is disabled, those benefits can continue to be paid into adulthood. To qualify for SSI benefits as an adult, an individual must be eligible as the child of someone who:

- is getting Social Security retirement or disability benefits
- has died and that child must have a disability that began prior to age 22

If a disabled child getting SSI turns 18 and continues to live with his or her parents, but does not pay for food or shelter, a lower SSI payment rate may apply.

For the autistic child who receives SSI benefits, turning 18 may have little effect on those benefits.

Entitlement Programs

55. Does autism usually qualify as a disability according to the Social Security Administration?

Historically, a child's diagnosis of autism was a guarantee of qualifying for supplemental security income payments, assuming the parents met the federal earnings and resources requirements. This evaluation is carried out by employees called Disability Examiners from the child's home state. In the past, these examiners simply looked at the diagnosis and approved the case. Things have changed since that idyllic time. The Social Security Administration (SSA) has imposed new changes and these changes have filtered down to the state Disability Determination Service (DDS) level. These changes mandate that the disability examiners look beyond the diagnosis and evaluate the functional ability of the child. According to the guide, the *Disability Evaluation under Social Security*, children must have "marked and severe functional limitations" in order to be found disabled.

The result of these changes is that a diagnosis of autism does not always guarantee an approval of benefits, although an evaluation of the child's disabilities within that diagnosis may.

For most children diagnosed with autism, meeting the requirement of marked and severe functional limitation should be easy if all their documentation and reports reflect their disabilities honestly.

Some problems that may result in an inappropriate benefits denial are:

- Evaluations and clinical reports that attempt to "spare the feelings" of the parents giving an inappropriately benign diagnosis or one that is purposely vague.
- Reports of clinical improvement under limited conditions, such as:
  - Within a limited time frame: For example, "the child's violent outbursts have decreased over the past 3 days" does not mean they are gone forever.
  - While with a particular teacher: Some teachers can exert better control over children or tend not to report poor behavior for other reasons.
  - While treated with a particular medication: Although a medication may make a real improvement, it is not necessarily sustained nor does it necessarily improve other behavior. For example, an antidepressant may improve a child's social withdrawal; however, it does not follow that an improvement will occur in his disabling tendency to wander or be inattentive in class.
- Variability in interpretation of the benefits eligibility standard:
  - The disability examiner alone determines disability.

- This determination is based on a personal definition of the terms used in the listings.
- Disability examiners may have little or no experience with the evaluation of autistic children.
- The disability evaluators are charged with interpreting the guidelines without adequate training in the subtleties of autism diagnosis and behaviors. For example, one of the biggest problems in the Social Security Listings for autism/PDD is found in Listing 112.10 A1b. It calls for the child to have "Qualitative deficits in verbal and nonverbal communication and in imaginative activity." Some disability evaluators may interpret this to mean that a profoundly retarded autistic child with behavioral problems that included violence and self-abuse would not be eligible for disability because one of the child's evaluations stated that the child appeared to have capacity for imaginative play.

Parents may be the only advocate a child has in this process. It is their duty to assure that their child gets the benefits they are entitled to. A fair decision can be made if accurate information is provided to the disability evaluator. Parents should see to the following:

- Make sure all physicians, psychologists, teachers, and therapists provide an honest and complete evaluation of the child.
- Their statements should show the full severity of the disability. The evaluations should report how the child behaves at a normal functioning level, not just when he or she is having a good day. Examples of the problem behavior should be included.
- Review the child's individual educational program (IEP) carefully. Make sure all the diagnoses are

Parents may be the only advocate a child has in this process.

139

correctly recorded and that a clear and comprehensive list of the child's disabilities is made.

- Review reports of behavioral or communicative improvements. Make sure they adequately reflect the conditions under which the behavior was observed, what conditions were required to achieve those improvements, and how long the improvement lasted (or was observed).

- Contest and demand clarification or revision on any evaluation that does not honestly reflect the child's ability.

56. What is Medicare?

Medicare

Title XVIII of the federal Social Security Act and 42 CFR 405 to 424; insurance-like payments for medical care of persons aged 65 and over; administered by federal Social Security Administration.

The **Medicare** program was created by Title XVIII of the Social Security Act. The program, which went into effect in 1966, was first administered by the Social Security Administration. In 1977, the Medicare program was transferred to the newly created Health Care Financing Administration (HCFA). HCFA has been renamed and is now called the **Centers for Medicare and Medicaid Services (CMS)**.

Centers for Medicare and Medicaid Services (CMS)

Formerly the Health Care Financing Administration; in the U.S. Department of Health and Human Services; the federal agency charged with overseeing and approving states' implementation and administration of the Medicaid program.

The CMS is a federal agency within the U.S. Department of Health and Human Services. CMS runs, among other programs, the Medicare and Medicaid programs, which are the two national health care programs that benefit about 75 million Americans. In 2003 CMS spent over $360 billion a year buying health care services for beneficiaries of Medicare, Medicaid, and the State Children's Health Insurance Program.

Medicare benefits are divided into two parts, creatively named Part A and Part B. Part A is called the hospital insurance program and it is funded by Social Security taxes. As one might expect from the name, Part A benefits pay for basic in-hospital services, extended care services, services provided in skilled nursing facilities, home health services, and hospice care for terminally ill patients. While in the hospital, the services covered include a semiprivate room, all meals, nursing services, hospital services, and supplies as well as the cost of inpatient mental health care with a lifetime limit of 190 days. Part A benefits are provided to eligible individuals at no personal expense.

Part B benefits help to pay for the costs of doctors' services, including office visits, but not routine physical exams. Medicare also covers outpatient medical and surgical services and supplies, any diagnostic tests, facility fees associated with approved procedures performed in an ambulatory surgery center, durable medical equipment (such as wheelchairs, walkers, etc.), second surgical opinions, outpatient mental health care, and outpatient occupational, physical, and speech therapy. As of 2004, Medicare beneficiaries are expected to pay a $100 annual deductible fee, 20 percent of the Medicare-approved amount, and 100 percent of charges above the approved amount as well as 50 percent of all outpatient mental health costs. Some Medicare coverage is available for approved medications.

57. What is Medicaid?

Medicaid is a national health insurance program aimed at serving the poor and the needy. All 50 states, the District of Columbia, Guam, Puerto Rico, and the U.S. Virgin Islands operate Medicaid plans. Medicaid was created by Title XIX of the Social Security Act and is part of the federal and state welfare system. State welfare or health departments usually operate the Medicaid program, within the guidelines issued by the CMS. The Medicaid program is funded by the general tax revenues of the federal and state governments. Persons covered by the Medicaid program have no out-of-pocket expenses for coverage.

Though Medicaid expenses can vary from state to state, the program must furnish the following services that are federally mandated:

- Inpatient hospital care
- Outpatient services
- Physician's services
- Skilled nursing home services for adults
- Laboratory and X-ray services
- Family planning services
- Early and periodic screening diagnosis and treatment for children under age 21

The eligibility requirements for Medicaid benefits are set by each state, although the CMS has set some minimum standards. The people who are eligible under these standards include the categorically needy and the medically needy.

The *categorically needy* are a group that includes families and certain children who qualify for public assistance. Therefore, they are eligible for Aid to Families with Dependent Children (AFDC) or Supplemental Security Income (SSI). Common examples of eligible persons include the aged, the blind, the physically or mentally disabled, and children.

The *medically needy* comprise a group who earn enough to meet their basic needs, but have inadequate resources to pay health care bills.

58. Is my autistic child eligible for Medicare or Medicaid benefits?

Your child can get Medicare coverage, but not immediately. Medicare is a federal health insurance program that was designed for people who are 65 or older and for people who have been getting Social Security disability benefits for at least 2 years.

Since children, even those with disabilities, do not get Social Security disability benefits until they turn 18, no child can get Medicare coverage until he or she is 20 years old.

The only exception to this rule is for children with chronic renal disease who need a kidney transplant or maintenance dialysis. Children with chronic renal disease can get Medicare if a parent is getting Social Security or has worked enough to be covered by Social Security.

Medicaid, by contrast, is a health care program for people with low incomes and limited assets. In most states, children who get SSI benefits qualify for Medicaid. In many states, Medicaid comes automatically with SSI eligibility. In other states, you must sign up for it. Some children can get Medicaid coverage even if they don't qualify for SSI. Check with your local Social Security office or your state or county social services office for more information.

59. What other health care services are available for my child?

State Children's Health Insurance Program (CHIP): Legislation passed in 1997 created a new Title XXI of the Social Security Act, known as the State Children's

Health Insurance Program (CHIP). This new program enables states to insure children from working families with incomes too high to qualify for Medicaid, but too low to afford private health insurance. The program provides protection for prescription drugs and vision, hearing, and mental health services and is available in all 50 states and the District of Columbia. Your state Medicaid agency can provide more information about CHIP or you can go to this Web site: cms.hhs.gov/schip/.

Children with Special Health Care Needs (CSHCN): If your child is disabled and is found to be eligible for SSI, he or she can be referred for health care services under the Children with Special Health Care Needs (CSHCN) provisions of the Social Security Act. These programs are generally administered through state health agencies.

Although there are differences from state to state, most CSHCN programs help provide specialized services through arrangements with clinics, private offices, hospital-based out- and inpatient treatment centers, or community agencies.

CSHCN programs are known in the states by a variety of names, including Children's Special Health Services, Children's Medical Services, and Handicapped Children's Program. Even if your child is not eligible for SSI, a CSHCN program may be able to help you. Local health departments, social services offices, or hospitals should be able to help you contact your CSHCN program.

Family Reimbursement Programs: These programs provide reimbursement for services not covered under other means such as Medicaid. Services reimbursed may include respite, camps, educational materials, therapies, and the like. Contact the Developmental Disabilities Council in your state for more information.

Entitlement Programs

PART VIII

Caring for Your Child After You're Gone

What is a will?

What is a special needs trust?

What is guardianship?

More . . .

60. I want to care for my child after I'm gone, but I was told by my lawyer not to leave any money in my child's name. Why is that?

In many states, money in your child's name can disqualify him or her from future state and federal financial aid. It may also trigger reclamation of past benefits that the child has received from the government, especially by Medicaid.

Before any money or other assets are left to your child with disabilities, you should first check with your legal or financial advisor. This may include any outright gifts of money or real estate or naming your child a direct beneficiary of your life insurance or retirement fund. If you have friends or family members who may want to give gifts to your disabled child, make sure these gifts do not result in more harm than good.

There are several ways to leave money for your child's care without disqualifying him or her from federal benefit programs. See the next section in this book on wills and **special needs** trusts.

61. Why does a parent with an autistic child need a will?

An autistic child may require supervision and financial support long after a parent has died. A well-written will can guarantee that your instructions will be known and followed after your death.

To die *intestate*—that is, without a will—places both your assets and your disabled child at risk. Without a will, your child could suffer great financial and emotional hardship, even if you know people who want to

Special needs

The unique, out-of-the-ordinary concerns created by a person's medical, physical, mental, or developmental condition or disability. Additional services are usually needed to help a person in one or more of the following areas: thinking, communication, movement, getting along with others, and taking care of self.

care for him or her and you have enough assets to see to his or her financial needs after you're gone. Without a will expressing your wishes, any of the following could occur:

- The distribution of your assets would be determined by an unknown judge in a probate court. This process could take months to resolve, and rather than having your assets distributed in accordance with your wishes, they are distributed in the way the court feels is appropriate.
- Your child could become a ward of the state. Courts would appoint a **guardian** who would be responsible for raising the child and administering any assets the child would receive from you or others.
- Your child could lose Medicaid benefits; then could be reduced to poverty through Medicaid reclamation. The state could go back years and demand repayment for past benefits, taking all or a portion of your child's inheritance.
- Your child could lose future Social Security benefits.
- Your adult (but disabled) offspring could be placed in charge of all your estate's assets and struggle to manage an inheritance he or she is unable to manage.
- Unscrupulous financial or legal "advisors" could take advantage of your child.

There is a lot to consider. To ensure the safety and protection of your child, consult a lawyer familiar with the needs of disabled children and make your wishes explicit in a written will.

62. What is a will?

A *will* is a written legal document that provides instructions for the disposition of your property (also called your assets or your estate) after you have died.

A well-written will can guarantee that your instructions will be known and followed after your death.

Guardian
An individual who has been entrusted by the law for the care of another person, for his or her estate (finances), or for both.

Caring for Your Child After You're Gone

The term "last will and testament" is simply a more complicated name for a will. A will is generally prepared with the help of an attorney.

A will is necessary for anyone who cares how their property is distributed upon their death, who would handle matters for those left behind, or who would serve as guardian for their minor children. The parents of an autistic child need to keep in mind that bequests made in a will can have an effect on their child's eligibility for federal benefits. If the disabled child is a direct beneficiary of money or other valuable assets with a value of greater than $2,000, this may disqualify the child from state and federal benefits.

When preparing a will, three people need to be identified within your will to make sure your wishes are carried out. These are the guardian, the trustee, and the executor.

- The *guardian* is a responsible adult whom you put in charge of caring for and raising your children who are less than 18 years old or any disabled adult child.
- The *trustee* is the person who will manage any property you wish to be held in a trust vehicle, usually for future use by beneficiaries.
- The *executor* for your estate is one who will be responsible for ensuring that all of your wishes as articulated in the will are carried out.

63. What is a special needs trust?

A special needs trust (also called a *supplemental needs trust*) is a legal vehicle that harbors assets for a disabled child or adult such that the resources are not considered in determining eligibility for government benefits. A special needs trust can be relatively inexpensive to establish and very often is a one-time investment.

Special needs trusts have become the planning tool of choice for many families of dependents with special needs. They can accomplish several goals that include:

- providing funds for the care of the individual with special needs without disqualifying him or her for government benefits
- keeping assets out of the child's name and control
- providing for the professional management of assets

A special needs trust is not like a regular trust fund. Mistakes made now in setting up the trust can be costly later. Therefore, although any attorney can set up a special needs trust, families should contact an attorney with experience in estate planning for those with developmental disabilities to set up such a trust for their child.

A special needs trust serves no purpose if there is not enough money in it to help your child when you're gone. Once the trust is established, parents, friends, and other family members can contribute to the trust. However, once the money is placed in the trust, it cannot be removed by the guardian or trustee, except for the specific benefit of the beneficiary. This limitation makes it common practice for parents and others to contribute little in the trust fund during their lifetime, since they may have unexpected needs for the money. Making the child's trust fund the beneficiary of bequests in the will or the beneficiary of a parent's life insurance policies, annuities, and qualified plans is now common. Finally, other family members and friends who want to help can put money into the trust.

A trustee's duties continue for the lifetime of the child.

64. Now that I have a trust, who should I choose to be trustee?

The trustee controls the assets placed in trust for the benefit of the special needs child. He or she responsible for distribution to the beneficiaries or for continued management of the assets. A trustee's duties continue for the lifetime of the child. A trust is a binding legal contract, so the trustee—whether a bank or a relative—has a legal obligation to follow your instructions and to manage the trust funds in a reasonable and prudent manner. Failure to do so can result in lawsuits by the child's guardian. The skills and financial acumen needed by the trustee depend on the size and type of assets in the trust. For larger trusts, the trustee may require expertise in collecting estate assets, investing money, paying bills, filing accountings (quarterly or annual), and managing money for beneficiaries. For more modest trusts, the trustee may only need to know what the needs of the child are and how to write a check.

The parents generally serve as trustee as long as they are alive. When they die, a successor trustee has to be ready to take over. The successor trustee, such as a family member or friend, can be named in the parent's or guardian's will. Because no individual lives forever, a bank or trust company should ultimately be designated as successor trustee.

The trustee should be selected for a number of qualities: financial discretion, knowledge of your loved one's special needs and likes and dislikes, as well as a genuine interest in the child's future. The biggest decision to make in designating a trustee is whether to use a family member or a professional. Although a lawyer or a banker can serve as trustee and may be skilled in financial matters, lawyers and banks are expensive and do not necessarily keep track of the disabled person's individual needs. If available, a responsible family member is usually a good choice.

65. What is a "letter of intent" and why is it necessary when creating a special needs trust?

A letter of intent is a written document that, although not legally binding, provides direction for the person or persons who will care for the child with special needs (the guardian) after the parents die or are no longer capable of caring for their child. Because it is not a legal document, it is a good idea for you to have it witnessed and notarized. If the child has cognitive ability, he should be involved in drafting the letter. The letter of intent helps the guardian or trustee to care for your child as you would. It should contain the parents' specific wishes and expectations, as they relate to the future of their disabled child. It is a working document for the future caregiver to follow. There is no regular format for a letter of intent, but it should be detailed and specific. The letter of intent should contain at least the following information about your child:

Medical history: The letter of intent should report any existing medical problems, any medications taken regularly, and any allergies to foods or medicines. All prior dental, surgical, or medical procedures should also be included. If you've had good experience with doctors or hospitals, put their names and contact information in this letter. Conversely, if you'd like to avoid certain physicians, therapists, clinics, or hospitals, state those wishes and the names of these providers in your letter of intent. Your child's physician should be able to help you with this.

Housing arrangements: Where should the child live? How long should they live there? Who should live with the child? Relatives? Friends? Do they need to live in a private or state institution or a particular adult home? Are there people you would not want your child to live with? Are there places or institutions you'd prefer your child to stay out of? How are the living arrangements to be paid for? The letter of intent is the place to write this information.

Education: What type of education would you like your child to get? What school should they attend? Should the child get vocational training? Religious instruction? How should the schooling be paid for?

Recreation and leisure activities: If your child loves to draw and paint and you want him or her to be able to continue to have art supplies and visit museums, this is the place to discuss that.

Legal papers: A description of the type and specific location of all legal papers that affect the child should be clearly recorded in this document. If the parents have a regular attorney, their name, address, and phone numbers should also be listed in this document. The names of your child's trustees, coguardians, or successor guardians also should be listed.

Child's personal preferences: Parents may be the only people who are familiar with the day-to-day things that make their child happy and comfortable. Therefore, the letter of intent should include general information and background about your child; such as their likes and dislikes regarding foods, favorite leisure activities, favorite toys, TV shows, sports, or video games. It should state the rights and values you want to preserve. Record the names of their circle of friends as well as professionals they are familiar with, including the dentist, barber, coach, music teacher, and so forth. If your daughter enjoys getting her hair styled or nails painted once a month, mention it here.

Religious preferences: The parents should be specific about what religion and religious services the child should participate in. How much religious instruction do you want your child to receive? Whom do you want to provide the instruction? Do you wish that they would attend religious services regularly? How often should it be: weekly, monthly, or yearly? Who should be responsible for transporting your child to services?

Final arrangements: In your letter of intent, describe any specific burial arrangements or religious services you'd like for your child.

66. What can a special needs trust pay for?

Federal benefit programs are designed to pay for the basic needs of their beneficiaries. Under SSI or Medicaid laws, basic needs means housing, food, and clothing. If the disabled person is receiving free housing, food, or clothing from someone else, including a family member or a trust, then the government benefits will be reduced or eliminated. Therefore, the money in a special needs trust cannot be used to pay for housing, food, or clothing.

The trust can pay for many things that will make your child's life more comfortable.

Despite this, the trust can pay for many things that will make your child's life more comfortable. Some things that the special needs trust can pay for are:

Home expenses: The trust *can* be used to purchase a home and perhaps rent it to the disabled person. The trust can pay for repairs, utilities, and taxes for a home; it can purchase furnishings for the home.

Recreation: The money that goes into these trusts can be used to enhance the life of your child over and above their medical care. It can pay for vacations, summer camp, or trips. It can buy recreational or sporting equipment for the child.

Other medical costs: Money in trust can be used to supplement or augment services that Medicaid does not cover, such as certain types of dental care, upgraded medical devices, extra or more intensive therapies, and vitamins.

End-of-life costs: It can pay for funeral and burial costs.

Legal costs: There are legal emergencies that a trust can pay for. If the person is not receiving the services needed from Social Security, Medicaid, or other government agencies, the trust can pay for an attorney or other advocate to fight for the individual. Without this type of help, the person might actually become homeless. If the disabled person is involved in an accident or is accused of a crime, the trust can pay for an attorney to defend them or look after their rights in a lawsuit.

67. Why do I need to establish guardianship for my adult child? Am I not his guardian already?

The subject of guardianship for a disabled child who is now an adult is of concern to most parents. Parents who have a child with a disability often assume that they can continue to be the legal guardian during the child's entire life. Although it may be obvious to a parent that their child does not have the capacity to make informed decisions, legally an adult is presumed competent unless otherwise deemed incompetent after a competency proceeding. In other words, while your son or daughter will always be your child, the courts will consider them an adult when reaching the age of 18. As an adult, your son or daughter may legally sign contracts, get credit cards, and borrow money. They can choose where to live, what doctors to see, and what surgery to undergo. Your adult child may dispose of their income and any savings that you have put in their name in any manner they choose or in any way that someone else convinces them. Most alarmingly, they may live with whomever they choose or marry without your consent or approval. The potential for acts of juvenile impulsiveness or for others to take advantage of your child is obvious.

68. What is guardianship?

Guardianship is a legal means of protecting children and adults who cannot take care of themselves, make decisions that are in their own best interest, or handle their assets. When the court determines that a person is incapable of handling either their personal and/or financial affairs and appoints a guardian, the person who is disabled is referred to as the guardian's *ward*. A guardian is responsible for monitoring the care of the ward. The guardian need not use their own money for the ward's expenses, provide daily supervision of the ward, or even live with the ward. However, the guardian must attempt to ensure that the ward is receiving proper care and supervision, and the guardian is responsible for decisions regarding most medical care, education, and vocational issues. For highly unusual decisions that were not anticipated at the time of the original guardianship hearing, the guardian should ask the court for instructions. The court must make decisions involving intrusive forms of treatment, such as administration of antipsychotic medication, sterilization, and the withdrawal of life-prolonging treatments. These unusual issues may be decided by parents and memorialized in their letter of intent for the care of their child. The court supervises guardianships; therefore, the guardian is required to report to the court annually on the status of the ward.

69. How do I obtain guardianship for my adult child?

If your child is not capable of caring for themselves or managing their finances, then you can seek a guardianship. However, just because you are the parent doesn't mean you are automatically named as guardian. You, like anyone else, must go through the legal system.

When establishing that your child is legally incompetent to care for themselves or manage their finances, your statement of their disabilities alone is not legally adequate. You will need to produce documentation of their diagnosis and associated disabilities. You may even need to pay to have their doctor testify in court or write affidavits concerning your child's medical condition and their capabilities.

Although obtaining guardianship is usually not a contentious issue, it can be time consuming and will cost money. To obtain guardianship, you need to hire an attorney and go to court. Be prepared for a complicated legal proceeding designed to protect your child's right to due process under the law. As with all guardianships, an attorney will be appointed to represent the rights of your child (the ward). A formal hearing will be held before a county judge to hear evidence whether your child is substantially unable to provide food, clothing, or shelter for themselves; to care for their physical health; or to manage their financial affairs. If so, the judge will appoint a guardian.

Because you are the one who is asking to be guardian, the court will appoint you (unless you are for some reason legally disqualified). At that point, you will have legal authority to make both monetary and medical decisions for your child. Equally important, your child's legal authority to manage funds will be terminated so that they cannot put the funds at risk. It often makes sense to name coguardians (for example, you and your spouse or you and another child) so if one dies or cannot continue for any reason, you have a backup without going through the court process all over again.

Many states allow the legal guardian to name a successor guardian. This is an important issue that should be discussed fully with both the successor guardian and your attorney. This declaration of guardianship can be

Many states allow the legal guardian to name a successor guardian.

contained in your will or in a separate legal document. When you die, the person named as the replacement guardian goes to court so the judge can appoint them as guardian (unless for some reason they are legally disqualified).

PART IX

Education of Autistic Children

What is the Individuals with
Disabilities Education Act?

What is special education?

How do I choose the best special education
program for my child?

More . . .

70. What does the Rehabilitation Act of 1973 have to do with the education of my child?

Accommodations

Changes in curriculum or instruction that do not substantially modify the requirements of the class or alter the content standards or benchmarks. Accommodations are determined by the individual education plan (IEP) team and are documented in the student IEP.

Americans with Disabilities Act (ADA)

A federal civil rights law passed in 1990. It prohibits discrimination on the basis of disability in (1) employment; (2) programs, services, and activities of state and local government agencies; and (3) goods, services, facilities, advantages, privileges, and accommodation of places of public accommodation.

As it turns out, this act has a lot to do with making **accommodations** for disabled children in schools. This act, specifically Section 504 of the act, is an important federal law for people with disabilities. Section 504 is a civil rights law. Its broad purpose is to protect disabled individuals from discrimination due to their disabilities. To be eligible for protection under section 504, a child must have a physical or mental impairment that substantially limits at least one major life activity. The **Americans with Disabilities Act (ADA)** is a similar document. It follows the format of section 504 but broadens the agencies that must comply with the rights and procedures outlined in section 504.

It is important to realize that section 504 and ADA do not guarantee direct special education services like those provided by the IDEA.

The law states that reasonable arrangements must be made for disabled students, but what are reasonable arrangements? Common accommodations made under section 504 or ADA include using assistive technology, removing obstacles to effective communications, and altering rules and policies. These accommodations may include granting children additional time for testing or allowing them to use other testing methods. Additionally, school personnel may change curriculum, materials, or architecture to meet the needs of a disabled student. Under section 504, if parents believe that their child has a disability, whether from autism or any other limitation, and the school system has reason to believe that the child needs special education or related services, the school is legally bound to evaluate the child to determine whether they are disabled as defined by section 504.

71. What is the Individuals with Disabilities Education Act, and why should I know about it?

Individuals with Disabilities Education Act (IDEA) is a federal law that establishes the educational rights of disabled children in the United States. It is one of the primary laws governing the education of children with disabilities. Becoming familiar with this law, its statutes, and regulations is important because it describes what services your child is entitled to and it gives parents a level playing field when discussing services and programs with local educators or committees on special education.

IDEA is a newer version of a law passed in 1975 called the Education for All Handicapped Children Act. IDEA was passed to further define the disabled child's rights to educational services as well as establish the role of the parent in the development of the educational plan for their child. IDEA has both statute and regulations: The statute is the governing legislation—the language of the law—and the regulations are an explanation of how the law is to be enacted.

IDEA regulations require the following:

- Duration of services. Your child may be eligible for services beyond the 180 days of a traditional school year.
- Identifying and evaluating the disability. Your child must be officially evaluated for having a disability

School personnel may change curriculum, materials, or architecture to meet the needs of a disabled student.

through specific testing procedures. Health, vision, hearing, social and emotional development, intelligence, communication skills, and academic performance must all be included during this evaluation.

- Free and appropriate education. The needs vary for each child with a disability but include education and related services. This is a comprehensive requirement that may include services such as transportation, psychological care, and physical therapy. Medical services are excluded from this provision.
  - The education costs for the disabled child will be borne by the state; the parents are not responsible for any of these costs. Although educational services are free, this does not mean they are the best services available. Some services beyond those minimally required may be available on a sliding price scale based upon family income.
  - IDEA insists on appropriate education for each child. However, the term "appropriate education" should not be construed to mean "best possible education" or "ideal education." The law merely establishes the minimal level of acceptable education and services that the state has to provide.

- **Least restrictive environment (LRE).** Handicapped children are mainstreamed into traditional classrooms with normally developing children whenever possible. Although this is not always feasible or appropriate, attempts should be made to limit a child's isolation.
- Individualized education program (IEP). Educational programs to fit specific needs are designed based upon the evaluation of a child's disability. Meetings are held with school personnel to identify goals and establish a program to help the child with available resources. The parents can participate in

---

Least restrictive environment (LRE)

A federal mandate that to the maximum extent appropriate, children with disabilities be educated with children who are not disabled. This means that the separation of children with disabilities from regular education buildings, programs, and students occurs only as much as necessary to meet the unique needs of special education students.

and contribute to these meetings and aid in the development of the educational plan.

- Early intervention services for infants and toddlers with physical, cognitive, communication, social or emotional, or adaptive developmental disabilities. This also may include infants or toddlers at risk for these developmental problems, depending upon the state.

- The educational goals and needed services will be established at least once a year in a document called the **individualized educational plan (IEP)**.

Copies of IDEA and its statutes and regulations are available from the government printing office or may be available at your public library. Detailed documentation of this law is also available on the following Web site: www.ed.gov/offices/OSERS/Policy/IDEA.

72. What is special education?

Special education can be defined as educational programming that is designed specifically for the individual student. This instruction is typically provided by the state at no cost to the parents. The instruction is specially designed to meet the unique educational needs of a student, with a goal of developing the student's maximum educational, social, and vocational potential.

Though the term special education is sometimes used to refer to programs for the intellectually gifted, most programs are developed to address the needs of the physically or mentally handicapped.

For the purposes of most school districts, handicapped students are those with the following conditions: learning disabled, speech pathology, visually impaired,

Individualized educational plan (IEP)

A team-developed, written program that identifies therapeutic and educational goals and objectives needed to appropriately address the educational needs of a school-aged student with a disability; a plan that identifies the student's specific learning expectations and outlines how the school will address these expectations through appropriate special education programs and services. It also identifies the methods by which the student's progress will be reviewed. For students 14 years or older, it must also contain a plan for the transition to postsecondary education, the workplace, or to help the student live as independently as possible in the community.

intellectually disabled, behavior disorders, autism spectrum disorders, hearing impaired, and physically impaired.

Common services provided for special education students include classroom instruction, physical education, and psychological and social work services. Speech, language, occupational, and physical therapies are also included.

Autistic children are not all the same. Each has unique strengths and weaknesses. What people with autism have in common is a developmental disability, a disorder of communication, which manifests itself differently in each person. Special education programs should be unique also.

Academic programs should begin with a full evaluation of the child's intellect and intellectual potential. Although it is true that some individuals with autism are below average in intelligence, many are above average. Therefore, academic programs should be individualized and academic goals need to be tailored to the individual's intellectual ability and functioning level. These programs should be flexible enough to accommodate a child's behavioral fluctuations and should be reevaluated on a regular basis.

Behavioral modification programs also must have unique goals based on an understanding of the child's past and current behaviors. For example, some children may need help in understanding social situations and developing appropriate responses. Others may exhibit aggressive or self-injurious behavior and need assistance managing their behaviors. No one program will meet the needs of all individuals with the disability, so it is important to find the program or programs that best fit the child's needs.

73. How do I get special education services for my child?

All U.S. children with disabilities are entitled to special education services under the regulations of IDEA law. To be eligible for special education services, the child's disability must first be objectively established. Disabilities are established either by an examination and report of independent physician qualified to make such a diagnosis or by a special education evaluation sponsored by the local educational agency. The evaluation can be undertaken when the child is first suspected of having a disability (preplacement evaluation) or when your child's level of functioning changes in one or more areas (reevaluation).

A child can be evaluated under the regulations of IDEA in two ways.

1. The parent can request an evaluation by calling or writing the director of special education or the principal of the child's home school.
2. The teachers or counselor in the school system who have observed the student may recommend an evaluation. The school system cannot mandate that a child undergo an educational evaluation and they must receive written permission from the parents before the evaluation can be conducted. Further, parents may refuse a school's request for a special education evaluation. However, the student cannot be enrolled in a special education class without an evaluation.

Evaluations are performed by a multidisciplinary team. The team is composed of specialist in the area of suspected disability (e.g., autism, mental retardation, or cerebral palsy) and at least one teacher. Parents may recommend professionals to the school for these evaluations. Though these professionals may be recognized experts in the evaluation and treatment of autism, the school is under no obligation to use them.

By law, the evaluation assesses many areas, including:

- General health
- Visual acuity
- Hearing
- Communication abilities
- Motor skills
- Learning abilities
- Social and/or emotional status

All of these areas are assessed and the results of each are taken into consideration when developing the child's educational program. No single area of disability can be used as the sole criterion for determining an appropriate education program for a child, according to IDEA regulations.

This evaluation becomes the basis for writing the child's individualized education program (IEP).

The individualized education plan (IEP) is a written legal document.

74. What is an IEP?

The individualized education plan (IEP) is a written legal document. This document is produced by the local district or department of education with the input and assistance of the parents (and, when appropriate, the student) after a thorough evaluation of the student's abilities and needs.

As the name implies, the educational program should be tailored to the unique needs of the student to achieve maximal educational benefit. These are not "one-size-fits-all" programs, not even among students with the same type of disability, such as autism. A program that is appropriate for one child with autism may be completely inappropriate for another.

The IEP should contain the following:

- A statement of the child's present level of educational performance. This should include both academic and nonacademic aspects of their performance (e.g., socialization interaction and aggressive behavior).
- A statement of **annual goals** that the student may reasonably accomplish in the next 12 months. This statement should also include a series of measurable, intermediate objectives for each goal. This will help both the parents and educators know whether the child is progressing and benefiting from their education.
- Appropriate objective criteria and evaluation procedures and schedules for determining, at least annually, whether the child is achieving the short-term objectives set out in the IEP.
- A description of all specific special education and related services, including individualized instruction and related supports and services, to be provided (e.g., occupational therapy, physical therapy, speech therapy, transportation, recreation). This includes the extent to which the child will participate in regular educational programs.

Annual goals
A set of general statements that represent expected achievement over a year's time for children with disabilities enrolled in special education programs and services. These are stated in the child's IEP.

- The initiation date and duration of each of the services, as determined, to be provided (this can include **extended school year services**).
- If your child is 16 years old or older, the IEP must include a description of transitional services (coordinated set of activities designed to assist the student in movement from school to post-school activities).

Extended school year services

Special education and related services provided to a qualified student with disabilities beyond the normal school year, in accordance with the student's IEP, and at no cost to the parent of the child. The need for extended services is determined by the student's IEP team.

As noted, the IEP provides the direction and goals that the teacher and therapist will work toward with the student. It describes how the teachers and therapists will measure those goals both during and at the end of the academic year. This allows parents and students to appreciate the progress in areas that might otherwise be invisible to them. This is why the IEP is known as the cornerstone for the education of a child with a disability.

As a legal document, the goals and selected services are not just a collection of hopes or wishes on how the school could educate a child. The school district or local educational agency is legally bound to educate your child in accordance with the IEP and may not change the academic goals or the services utilized because they are difficult or expensive to undertake.

75. What can I do if I don't agree with the findings in the IEP?

It is common for parents and educational agencies to have a legitimate difference of opinion regarding the student's placement, educational goals, or need for special services. This difference of opinion may stem either from a school's lack of appreciation of the student's needs (that the parent is keenly aware of) or from a parent's unfamiliarity with the scope and limitations of special services. If these misunderstandings cannot be resolved at the IEP meeting, the parents have recourse in the law.

Within the law, there are specific procedural safeguards to protect the child's rights. If parents disagree with the local educational agency, they can seek redress in the following ways:

- *Discussion of the child's needs with knowledgeable experts.* An informal discussion with objective experts can help to educate the parents about what the child needs in the way of education and special services. Experts may include educators or counselors in or outside of the school. Further, the parents may want to discuss their child's needs and IEP determinations with physicians, psychologists, developmental neurologists, or a lawyer. This type of discussion may result in the parents appreciating the wisdom of the IEP findings or may encourage them to proceed with their complaints.
- *IEP review.* Parents, at any time, may request that the educational agency review the IEP findings and take into account the parents' concerns and any new information available.
- *Complaint resolution.* Educational agencies are required to publish and adhere to a complaint resolution procedure. Parents and other advocates may file a complaint with the educational agency. The parents' complaint about IEP usually alleges that the educational agency has denied a student's rights for special educational services under IDEA. By federal law, the state educational agency must resolve the issues of the complaint within 60 calendar days after it is filed.
- *Mediation.* The parents and educational agency may engage in nonbinding mediation to resolve the dispute according to IDEA. The cost of the mediation

process is borne by the state; participation in the mediation process is voluntary and neither party is bound to accept the resolution that is recommended by the mediator. Mediation sessions are conducted by a neutral third person (mediator) who assists the parents and the school agency in resolving their dispute. To meet the requirements of IDEA, all states must have an established mediation process.

- *Due-process hearing.* Parents may request a due-process hearing if they disagree with the findings of the IEP. The due-process hearing is a legal proceeding, the findings of which are binding. Parents and other advocates may benefit from professional legal advice.

William's comment:

We had an unfortunate experience with our local school district. Several months after our initial IEP, we received word that we would be unable to continue using the same ABA program for our son. The alternatives they suggested weren't adequate. Not even close. We consulted a lawyer. He informed us that the school district couldn't disallow the program and that there were problems with the format and goals of Liam's IEP. We spent some time and money but we were able to resolve these problems to our satisfaction.

We fought it and won. We wound up getting more hours and a longer calendar year for services. The school districts wanted to save money and limit services at the expense of our child. They even sent a "district specialist" who tried to make a deal for lesser services with us BEFORE we went to mediation. They talk a big game, but in my experience, the last thing a district wants to do is go to a hearing. Bottom line: Don't be afraid to fight these people.

If parents or guardians are unsure of their rights under the IDEA, they can contact the U.S. Department of Education's Office of Special Education Programs. OSEP will provide parents and other interested parties with information or clarification on education rights. The OSEP can be contacted at:

The Office of Special Education Programs
U.S. Department of Education
400 Maryland Avenue SW
Mail Stop 2651
Washington, DC 20202
202-205-5507
www.ed.gov/offices/OSERS/OSEP/index.html

William's comment:

We see a major problem with services available for diagnosed kids. There are nowhere near enough qualified service providers. As far as individualized education plans that are required by law for children with special educational needs, we have found that the school districts often put their agenda ahead of the child in need. They seem prone to recommending treatment that isn't much more than putting a bandage over a bullet wound or justifying the inadequacies of their own infrastructure by putting unqualified educators on a child's case. Our experiences lead us to believe that the special needs child is not the first concern of the district.

76. How do I choose the best special education program for my child?

There is no single best special education school or program for all children with autism. The ideal program

Parents can improve the chance of getting the best program by doing some research beforehand.

for your child is closely matched to their unique abilities and interests. However, life is rarely ideal and there are always limitations in getting the best type of treatment for your child. These limitations include the availability of schools that have programs and therapists in your area, the flexibility of this program to accommodate your child's needs, the geographic convenience of getting to that program, and the financial cost of the program.

Parents can improve the chance of getting the best program by doing some research beforehand. Before making decisions on your child's treatment, you will want to gather information about your child's needs, abilities, and interests as well as information about local and regional schools and the programs in those schools. Your child's needs and abilities are evaluated by the local school district or educational provider and are explained in the IEP. If you are unfamiliar with any of the technical terms or meaning of the conclusions, you are entitled to have them fully explained to you. You should keep a copy of the IEP with you when visiting a school, so that you can discuss its contents with the teachers and therapist at the prospective programs.

Before evaluating the schools, parents should keep in mind that an effective special education program for autistic children has the following characteristics:

- Encourages early intervention in the child's behavior
- Is highly structured
- Has a predictable schedule with a stable staff of teachers and therapists
- Specialized programs with qualified therapists (speech, physical, music, etc.)
- Has a low student-to-teacher ratio

- Tasks are taught as a series of simple steps
- Teachers and therapists make an effort to actively engage the child's attention
- Understands and builds on the child's interests
- Provides regular and consistent positive reinforcement of appropriate behavior
- Encourages parental involvement in the therapy and continuation of the therapy at home

You can learn more about the available programs in your area by comparing the qualities just noted against the advertised qualities of the local programs. Additional information can be gained by asking questions of the special education teachers in the area or by consulting with members of the local autism society or parent's support group. Visiting the schools themselves is an excellent way to gather information about class size, student-to-teacher ratio, and staff turnover as well as specific information about the therapies and the qualification of the therapists employed. When speaking with a teacher or administrator from a special education program, a parent shouldn't be afraid to ask some of the following questions:

- Is this program based on sound, scientific principles? What are they?
- Is this program or any of the therapies in it considered experimental? (It is best to avoid experimental programs.)
- Are the teachers and therapists in this program qualified, certified, and licensed?
- Does this program treat all aspects of autism or just some?
- How much money, time, and effort does the program require of the parents or guardians? (Parents may not have the time or resources to devote to an

intensive program because of other children or work commitments.)

- Is the program open to all children with autism? Are there any limitations regarding age or abilities? For example, can the program accommodate an autistic child who is high functioning? In a wheelchair? Is 19 years old? Is also deaf?

After examining all the options, you can make the best decision about your child's treatment based on your child's needs and the available resources.

77. Are computers useful in the education of an autistic child?

Yes, computers are a useful adjunct to any educational program for autistic children, whether school based or home based. Computers can be an ideal environment for promoting communication, social development, creativity, and playfulness for individuals even at the extreme of the autistic spectrum. Well-designed computer software is interesting, responsive, interactive, and presented in more than one mode (i.e., visual and auditory). Beyond this, computers have other attributes that make them ideal tools for autistic children. These attributes include:

- *Computers are consistent.* A computer running appropriate software is consistent in its responses, more so than any parent or teacher could ever hope to be. Further, if the computer is functioning well, it will deliver no unwanted surprises to the child.
- *Computers are "patient."* Computer programs, unlike parents or teachers, do not chafe with repeated demands of the autistic child. They will happily answer the same question a hundred times or tell the same story a thousand times.

- *Computers are nonjudgmental.* Children can make errors safely within the context of the programs and are not subject to the admonishments or uncomfortable redirection of teachers or parents.
- *Computers are safe.* A properly supervised child will neither be harmed nor frightened by the computer.
- *Computers are empowering.* Experience has shown that many children with autism like to use the computer because it is a safe, structured, predictable environment. The child has complete control over the computer and the environment created on the computer screen. Autistic children seldom feel in control of their environment and working with a computer can allow them to experience this positive and calming sensation.
- *Computers can accommodate a child's communication style.* Communication deficits are a hallmark of autism. Computers allow the autistic child to interact with the software program through several non-verbal modalities including the key-board, mouse, and touch-screen. For children with physical disabilities, computers can be equipped with voice recognition software such that the computer responds to a limited number of voice commands or equipment that responds to visual gaze or chin stick.
- *Computers are fun and instructive.* Autistic children, like typical children, enjoy using the computer. Programs that might be viewed as "games" are used as tools for learning sequence, cause and effect, and manipulation of environment. Good software programs incorporate music, color, and loveable characters to tell stories, identify shapes, or teach math and vocabulary. The children's attraction to the computer is often strong enough that teachers can use educational software programs in the classroom as a reward for good behavior.

William's comment:

Our child's biggest challenge is his ability to socialize appropriately. Though it seems counterintuitive, we use video games to encourage socialization. Liam loves his video games, and so we use video games as a reward and reinforcer for his therapy. When he makes eye contact, addresses others, or shares appropriately, he is allowed some time on his video game. It is our hope that in the future, it will be something that will serve as a common interest between him and his friends. Video games hopefully will give him a reason to want to interact with his peers.

78. What type of computer should an autistic child use?

Computers are machines that have both hardware and software. The hardware consists of those things that you can touch and feel, such as the monitor (or screen), the central processing unit, the keyboard, and the mouse. The software (also known as a computer program) is what makes the computer hardware operate. It is composed of the operating system as well as the games and other interactive learning tools.

Hardware: A basic computer system should include enough computer memory and processing speed to operate the software you purchase for your child. It should also have a monitor, keyboard, mouse, and speakers. Although laptop computers offer the advantage of portability and easy storage, they are also easily, lost, dropped, or broken. A desktop computer is larger, but is easier to secure on a flat surface. In addition, its sensitive parts, such as the central processing unit, can be placed on the floor while the monitor and keyboard can be placed on a desk or table. This decreases the chance of the computer being dropped and damaged. If you are planning to purchase a computer for your child, first discuss your child's needs with the computer salesperson or consultant before purchasing the computer. This will prevent you from purchasing either a computer system that is inadequate to your needs or one that is overequipped or overly expensive.

We just ordered a children's mouse that is less sensitive and easier to manage for his little hands.

Software: The type of software your child should use depends upon what goal you have for your child. Some software programs have been designed for typical children and some have been designed specifically for autistic children. They are designed to elicit math and language development, cognitive development, or just for play. Generally, any software can be used if a child shows interest. Some Web sites of organizations that focus on autism will list software titles that have been used successfully with children with autism.

Some attributes that a parent should look for in the software program include:

- The program is easy to install and use for both parents and children.
- The program is designed to teach concepts as well as facts. For example, fire is dangerous rather than "you shouldn't touch matches."
- Programs help teach self-awareness, a concept difficult for children with autism.
- The software is developed to work for children with few receptive language skills.
- Programs demonstrate and encourage appropriate behavior for children with autism (for example, no

Any software can be used if a child shows an interest in it.

hitting, no wandering, and wash your hands after using the bathroom).

Generally, any software can be used if a child shows an interest in it. Software designed specifically for autistic children may not be necessary for your child. Some places to look for educational software include:

Laureate Learning Systems: A catalogue of educational tools, books, flashcards, and computer programs; www.laureatefamily.com

Diff Roads to Learning: A resource for educational ABA materials for children with autism; www.difflearn.com

Help for Asperger's Kids: An activity book that teaches critical social skills; www.InstantHelpBooks.com

Autism and Computing: A not-for-profit group, its aim is to explore ways of minimizing the effects of autism; www.autismandcomputing.org.uk/index.en.html

Computhera: Offers a seven-step gradual discrete approach for teaching reading to autistic children; www.computhera.com

79. When discussing plans for my teenage son, I've heard the term "transition." What does it mean?

As an autistic child reaches the late teens, their entitlement to public education ends, as does the security of federally mandated services. For many autistic children, this is a time of transition from school life to adult life, making it one of the most challenging times for individuals with autism and their families. It is a time to address questions about continued education, vocational training, and employability. For students with disabilities, these choices are more difficult to make and require a great deal of planning.

Despite the difficulty associated with this planning, the issues surrounding this transition period should not come as a surprise to most parents with autistic children. They will have been planning for this transition for 4 or more years. While entitlement to public education ends at 18, federal law (IDEA) requires that transition planning begin at 14, becoming a formal part of the student's IEP. Transition planning should involve the student, parents, and members of the IEP team who work together to help the individual make decisions about their path.

Transition services are provided by the local public school or educational provider. They are intended to prepare students to make the transition from the world of the student to the world of adulthood. The IEP team reviews all of the child's evaluations to gain insight into their abilities, assets, and interests before they can determine what types of transition services a student needs. They must consider the appropriateness of the child for such areas such as continued academic education, vocational training, employment, independent living, and community participation.

Transition services are a coordinated set of activities that are based on the student's needs and that take into

Transition services
A coordinated set of activities that promote movement from school to postschool education, vocational training, integrated employment (including supported employment), continuing and adult education, adult services, independent living, or community participation. Transition goals are determined by the IEP team beginning at age 14 and are based on student and family vision, preferences, and interests.

account their preferences and interests. Transition services can include instruction, community experiences, the development of employment and other postschool adult living objectives, and (if appropriate) the acquisition of daily living skills and functional vocational assessment. The transition team is not just composed of members of the special education team. The student and family are expected to take an active role in the planning.

PART X

Living with Autism

What are some tips for parenting
kids with autism?

How can I help my other children form a
relationship with their autistic sibling?

How do I make my home safe
for my autistic child?

More . . .

Having a child diagnosed with autism is a devastating blow to parents.

80. My child was just diagnosed with autism. What do I do first?

Having a child diagnosed with autism is a devastating blow to parents. Even the most well-informed parent will find themselves shocked and at a loss for what to do. If you feel this way, don't be alarmed. It is as natural as it is painful. There are things to do, so start making a list. It will make you feel better and will help your child. Start with this:

Confirm the diagnosis. Autism can be mistaken for other diseases, so before treatment begins, parents should be certain that their child has autism. Parents should ask themselves that following questions:

- Did a doctor make the diagnosis?
- Was the doctor qualified to make the diagnosis?
- Does the doctor have training and experience on the diagnosis of children with developmental diseases?
- Has the doctor ruled out other diseases that can be mistaken for autism such as a hearing impairment, ADD/ADHD, genetic disorders, and mental retardation?

If the answer to any of these questions was "no," the parents may want to have the child evaluated by a multispecialty team with expertise in the diagnosis of developmental disorders.

Seek appropriate care for your child. Find the local early intervention program. Discuss the attributes of the program with experts. For example, you may want to ask about what services and therapies are provided and what the student-teacher ratio is. Enroll your child in an early intervention program as soon as possible. It should provide speech, physical, and occupational therapy.

William's comment:

Do not procrastinate, get right on it. The earlier the intervention, the better for everyone involved.

Educate yourself. Begin reading about the topics of autism, autism behaviors, diseases associated with autism, special education, early intervention programs, federal educational entitlements, and behavioral treatment programs. Many articles, books, and Web sites are available for this purpose. Also helpful is contacting the local chapter of the Autism Society of America. Attend a meeting of this chapter and subscribe to their newsletter. Find parents in your area who have an autistic child and who have been dealing with this issue longer than you. They can provide you with insights, information, and support.

Develop a support network. Do not keep your child's diagnosis a secret. Tell your friends and family and solicit their help and support. Keep in mind that caring for an autistic child is more like a marathon than a sprint. Though you may have the time and energy now, you have to consider what you will require in the future or if your current situation changes. Families that cope well with the stress of a newly diagnosed autistic child are able to identify their needs and ask for help. This help can range from babysitting to transportation, from the social to the psychological.

William's comment:

We don't have any of our family near where we live and that makes it hard. I have no doubt this road would be easier if we had family members around to support us.

Discuss your child's diagnosis with your lawyer. You may need your attorney's help if getting educational entitlements for your child proves difficult. Your attorney may also want to discuss such issues as life insurance, your estate, wills, trusts, and guardianship with you, because they can have an impact on your child.

Consider counseling for yourself, your spouse, and your children. The diagnosis of autism can be psychologically devastating for parents and the demands of caring for an autistic child can be exhausting. These pressures can put a strain on many people in the family. If so, discussing the situation with a psychologist, psychiatrist, family counselor, or clergy member may be helpful.

Avoid "snake oil" salespeople. Unfortunately, there is no known cure for autism. Anyone who promises a cure should be avoided. Parents of recently diagnosed children are emotionally vulnerable and have been taken advantage of by unscrupulous practitioners. Parents should be cautious before investing any amount of money in an unknown or unproven treatment. Effective interventions that can improve autistic behavior do exist and are available through a qualified special education program. Using diet and vitamins or other alternative therapies are not helpful in the majority of cases. Spend your time, money, and emotional energy on proven treatments such as intensive behavioral therapy.

Avoid feeling guilty about your child's autism. Parents cannot cause autism. The cause of autism remains unknown, but what we do know is that some theories about the causes of autism, theories that have been popular in the past, have been disproved. These disproved theories include: autism is caused by bad mothering, autism is caused by food allergies, and autism is caused by vaccinations.

This is easier said than done. A conscious effort has to be made to remind yourself that there is nothing that you did that caused the autism in your child.

81. What are some tips for parenting kids with autism?

For the parent whose child is newly diagnosed, the following are tips to help you avoid pitfalls in dealing with your child.

Pay attention to your child's environment and routine.

- Keep the environment predictable and familiar.
  - Have a regular schedule that the household follows and post it on the refrigerator or other obvious place.
- Prepare your child for changes.
  - Use pictures and calendars to help your child predict upcoming events.
    - Clearly mark on the calendar when a trip to the dentist or pediatrician will occur.
    - Explain what will happen and promise a reward for good behavior.
    - There are many children's books on topics such as trips to the dentist, doctor, or grandma's house that can be read and explained to a child in anticipation of the first visit.
  - When moving your child from an activity that they enjoy to another activity, give them a "countdown." A countdown lets a child know they will have to change activities in a few minutes. For example, "15 minutes and the TV goes off" or "30 minutes till bedtime." Then mention the change in activity every few minutes until the activity changes. Using an egg timer or alarm clock is

helpful for reinforcement. The countdown approach significantly decreases tantrums.

- Provide structure and routine.
  - Autistic children require structure and routine and can become quite upset when even small changes occur.
  - Create a daily list of events with required activities for the child.
    - This daily list can be photocopied and used every day.
    - Allow the child to check off accomplished activities.
    - In addition to such things as playtime and bedtime, the daily list of activities should include required chores, homework, bathing, and grooming activities. In this way, the list of daily activities not only provides a calming reference for the child, but reinforces appropriate behaviors.
  - Making sure that daily routines are not interrupted unnecessarily will reduce a child's fear and anxiety as well as unwanted behavior.
    - Continue the routine as much as possible when traveling with your child.
    - Make sure babysitters or respite providers are made aware of the list of daily activities and whatever rewards are attendant to good behavior. This will make the babysitter's job easier and ease the child's anxiety.
- Be aware of sensory stimuli from the environment. It can upset the child and affect behavior. Some examples are:
  - *Noise*: This can be as obvious as construction sounds from the street or as subtle as the buzzing from a fluorescent light or rush of air from the air conditioning duct. Be aware of any changes and modify them when appropriate.

Be aware of sensory stimuli from the environment.

- *Temperature*: When possible, control the temperature of the child's bedroom and play space. Be aware that some medications, such as neuroleptics or sulfa drugs, can make the child more sensitive to excess heat or sun exposure.
- *Smells*: Some smells bother autistic children. Be aware of new smells in the environment. These include cleaning products, paints, solvents, glues, perfumes, and deodorants. When possible, use cleaning products while your child is at school and move the child's bed to your bedroom or the basement when painting his room.
- *Strange people*: Autistic children can get excited or withdrawn in the presence of new people.
  - When possible, let autistic children know when a friend or relative will come to visit.
  - When possible, post a picture of the visitor on the refrigerator for the child to see. Refer to it frequently before the visit.
  - Prepare them for visits to doctor's or dentist's offices or visits to the barber by telling them what will happen, calming their fears, and promising rewards for good behavior.

When you talk to your child:

- Speak clearly and in complete sentences.
- When giving instructions, be as organized and concise as possible.
- Avoid rhetorical questions or sarcastic statements. They're not likely to be understood and will increase the tendency of the child to ignore speech.
- Avoid discussion of abstract concepts. When possible, speak in concrete terms.
- Try to respond consistently to a child's questions or other attempts at communication.

- Ignoring a child's attempts at communication discourages him or her and reinforces the tendency for withdrawal.

To help your child improve his or her behavior:

- Help your child learn to communicate.
  - Work on communication early and frequently.
  - Be consistent in your efforts. It will help your child improve.
  - Better communication will help relieve your child's frustration and may lead to better behavior.
  - Model simple phrases for your child, such as "may I have . . ." or "I want. . ." Have your child repeat the phrase before accommodating their request.
  - Use gestures, sign language, picture boards, and communication devices when speech is not possible.
- Teach your child to make choices.
  - An inability to decide or make choices is a characteristic of autism.
  - Providing opportunities to make choices every day may help with this. Some choices that you can provide your child with are what clothes to wear, what game to play, what channel to watch, or what snack to eat.
- Be consistent in rewarding positive behavior.
  - Identify positive behavior that you'd like your child to emulate.
  - Reward the behavior every time and as immediately as possible.
  - Rewards may consist of verbal praise, a star on their daily list of accomplishments, or a snack or toy.
- Unwanted behavior should be identified early and addressed immediately.

- Consistently address unwanted behavior; don't let some bad behavior slide. Not addressing bad behavior will guarantee that it will be repeated.
- Autistic children often cannot "read" emotional signals such as an angry tone of voice or angry facial expression. Therefore, gain your child's attention and let them know what behavior you expect in clear and concise terms.
- Replace the unwanted behavior with a favorite activity; that is, use distraction.
- While denying a reward in response to unwanted behavior is appropriate, physical punishment is not likely to encourage good behavior and is not recommended.
- Choose rewards you know your child will like and that you can provide.
  - Promising a particular reward for a good behavior and not being able to provide it immediately after your child has accomplished the specific task is a common mistake. Tantrums and a missed opportunity to reinforce good behavior are the unfortunate outcomes.
- Before a particular reward is promised:
  - Purchase any toys or snacks that you will use as a reward before you promise them.
  - Call the park, pool, arcade, or movie theater to make sure they're open before promising a trip.

82. Traveling with my autistic child is difficult. What can I do to make "going out" easier?

Yes, traveling with an autistic child can be difficult. Taking an autistic child out of their rigid social routine is uncomfortable. Going to new places and meeting strangers can be frightening. Boats, bus and train stations, and airports can overwhelm the child with sensory stimuli. Consider the gauntlet of security, identity papers, interrogators, metal detectors, and baggage X-ray machines the average airport puts their customers through.

Dr. Quinn's comment:

I find this overwhelming at times and know that it frightens our autistic son.

Nevertheless, with preparation, many parents are able to travel with their autistic children comfortably.

Some suggestions to make travel more comfortable are:

Decrease the amount of stimulation when possible.

- When possible, travel at times when the public conveyances are least crowded.
- Start car trips in the early morning, so that the child can sleep for the first few hours of a long trip.
- When eating out or shopping, try to choose nonbusy times or off-peak hours.

Try to avoid delays and unanticipated waiting time.

Nevertheless, with preparation, many parents are able to travel with their autistic children comfortably.

- Book the first appointment when visiting the doctor or dentist so that your child does not have to sit for too long in the waiting room.
- Be the first or last patron at the barber or stylist.
- At the airport, train, or bus terminal, notify gate personnel that you are traveling with a disabled child and request that you are first on the bus, train, or airplane. This will prevent a long wait and get you seated quickly.
- Many amusement parks will allow disabled children (and accompanying adult) to go to the head of

the line. For example, Disney World has a guest assistance card or special guest pass for children with disabilities. This pass allows them access to rides without long waits or to go to the front rows of the theater.

Avoid, when possible, visiting places that require the utmost decorum and restrained behavior from children.

- Choose "family" restaurants or chain restaurants that don't expect perfect behavior from young patrons.
- Visiting a zoo rather than a museum is a better choice till your child becomes comfortable with traveling and visiting new places.

Anticipate difficulties and plan ahead.

- Call ahead to make sure that site is open for business *before* telling your child that you are going somewhere. This will prevent disappointment and a classic "parking-lot tantrum."
- Before embarking on long trips, be sure to have an alternate plan or destination to entertain or distract your child in case problems arise. This might include the timing of the arrival, traffic, weather, or an unplanned closing.
- In airports and other places where security guards are charged with interrogating and detaining suspicious people, notify them in advance that your child is mentally disabled. Left unexplained, the behaviors and characteristics of an autistic child may delay your trip and cause unnecessary anxiety. Encounters with uninformed security guards are the types of situations that can easily escalate into misinterpretations, verbal and physical confrontations, physical containment, and restraint.

- Take books, pens, and toys for your child to play with to occupy idle time.
- When possible, have another adult accompany you. This may be invaluable for such minor emergencies as trips to the men's room if you are a woman, another set of hands to move a reluctant child from a toy display, or freeing one adult to ask directions while the other entertains the child.
- When away on vacation or extended trip, try to observe the usual daily routine as much as possible.
  - Have your child complete the usual activities of work, play, and bedtime.
  - Try to keep your child's environment as familiar as possible by taking your child's favorite toy, video game, bed covers, or bedside lamp. This will make strange environments easier to handle.

William's comment:

What the refrigerator did for meat products, the portable DVD player did for parents of autistic kids! This small device can keep our boy cool for extended trips (in the car or on the plane). Wow! Moreover, they're getting lighter, smaller, and much cheaper.

Traveling with an autistic child can be stressful to the child and the parent. By preparing well and spending time reinforcing good behavior with plenty of rewards (such as verbal praise and small gifts such as candy or toys), the next trip can be made much easier.

83. Keeping my child clean and neat is a real challenge. How do other parents deal with this?

A common complaint among parents of autistic children is the difficulty in getting their child to bathe, brush his teeth, and perform even basic grooming. Although not unheard of among typical children, this behavior is intensified in the autistic population. An autistic child's tendencies to avoid noisy environments, close contact with other people, and tactile stimulation make personal hygiene difficult. Autistic children find the bright lights and loud noises in tiled bathrooms, difficult to tolerate. Similarly, the close physical contact, noise, and strangeness of a barber shop are equally difficult. Despite this, most parents are able to achieve acceptable levels of hygiene and grooming in their children. Like other behavioral challenges in autistic children, it requires equal measures of resourcefulness, discipline, and compromise from the parents.

Despite this, most parents are able to achieve acceptable levels of hygiene and grooming in their children.

Living with Autism

Some suggestions include:

- Extremely high levels of cleanliness may be inappropriate or simply too difficult to achieve. There is no medical reason to bathe your child daily. If your child resists bathing, aim for one or two baths per week.
- Explore alternatives to daily bathing or showering. Consider sponge baths or washing him or her with a damp cloth while he or she watches television or plays a video game.
- **Discrete trials** that are aimed at desensitizing the child to the water in a bath or shower can be effective. Using the novelty of jumping into swimming pools, playing in outdoor showers, or jumping over lawn sprinklers may help the child overcome their fear of water.
- For some children cutting the finger and toenails is frightening or unpleasant because of its strangeness. Parents can try to cut their child's nails when they are distracted with a TV program or video game or

Discrete trial

A short, instructional exercise that has three distinct parts: e.g., a direction, a behavior, and a consequence.

even when they're asleep. Alternatively, a parent could try teaching them to do it themselves.

- If your child is sensitive to getting his or her hair cut at the hairdressers, try hugging him or her in your lap. Regularly brushing your child's hair may "desensitize" him or her to getting his or her hair cut. If the child is frightened by the noise of an electric clipper or hair dryer, ask the barber or stylist to only use scissors and a comb and to let the hair dry naturally.

84. Getting (and keeping) my child dressed is very difficult. What can I do to make it easier?

For many autistic children, wearing clothes is an uncomfortable proposition, and it is common for them to tend to take their clothes off whenever they can. Some clothes present an overwhelming **tactile** stimulation to the autistic child and while their desire to remove their clothes is understandable, it can be socially inappropriate for them and embarrassing for their parents. Some suggestions for avoiding these situations are:

Tactile

Related to the sense of touch.

- Make sure they have comfortable clothes on.
  - Ask your child why they want to take their clothes off. They may be able to tell you what's irritating them.
  - Choose soft fabrics, preferably cotton.
  - Check clothes for thick or rough seams that may irritate skin before you purchase them.
  - Avoid clothing with tight waistbands, collars, or cuffs.
  - Remove clothing tags that may rub against their skin.

- When the children are older, allow them to pick out the clothes they want to wear for the next day. Try to determine why some clothes are chosen and not others.
- Remember, your child also may be sensitive to the color or pattern of the clothes.
- If keeping a diaper on is difficult, make sure it is not on too tight. Change brands to find one whose texture is the least irritating. This may take some time.
- If communication is difficult or the child is too young to work with, try dressing them in clothes that are difficult to remove.
  - Select overalls or jumpsuits.
  - Choose shirts, dresses, and pants that button at the back.
  - Replace zippers, Velcro, buttons, and other easily opened fasteners with more complicated options.
- Your child may be overly sensitive to the feeling of clothes against their skin. Consult with your occupational therapist for help to develop a "desensitization" program.
- Be aware of other issues that may cause the child to want to remove their clothes.
  - Are the clothes too warm for the temperature or activity level?
  - Are they too restrictive for the type of play?
  - Does your child have an allergy to the cloth or detergents used to clean it?
  - Does your child have a skin rash, such as eczema or a sunburn that is irritating?
  - Does your child have an infection from parasites such as pinworms, ticks, body lice, or scabies? This is not an unusual finding, especially in children that attend special education classes with

other developmentally disabled students. Consult
your pediatrician if suspicious.

- Provide reinforcement to the child for proper
behavior.
  - Praise the child effusively for wearing appropriate
  clothes.
  - When dressed in a new outfit, have your child
  look in the mirror; they may like what they see.
  - Point out that siblings and parents wear clothes;
  autism does not eliminate a child's desire to dress
  like an adult.

85. What are some causes of behavioral change in autistic children?

Behavioral problems in autistic children can range from
difficulty with transitioning from task to task, associated with uncooperativeness or defiance to aggression,
uncontrollable tantrums, and self-abusive behavior,
such as biting of the hands and arms. These behaviors are recognized as part of autism and can be expected to wax and wane over time. Exacerbations of
behavior are sometimes easily attributed to changes in
the environment, encountering strangers, or having
new demands placed on the child at school or at home.
Sometimes the behaviors have no identifiable cause
and must be tolerated as part of the disease. Before a
worsening of behavior or new behaviors can be attributed to "being autistic," parents, teachers, and
physicians must be aware of other causes that may
be serious. Because communication is a problem
with autistic children and adults, they may find it difficult to tell their caregivers that they are feeling sick
or are in pain, irritated, or frightened. This frustration, caused by an inability to communicate, may man-

ifest itself as aggression or self-injury. Alternatively, severe pain, nausea, or weakness may make the child withdraw and not participate in play or school. Behavioral problems can escalate in these situations, especially if the child is pressured to continue with daily routine or work activities.

Some things parents should look out for are:

Infection. Parents and caregivers should be vigilant for illnesses that can be the cause of behavioral changes, even changes that occur slowly and are sometimes dismissed as typical autistic behavior. When a child has a deterioration of behavior, parents or caregivers should consider influenza, sore throats, ear infections, tooth abscesses, migraine headaches, abdominal pain, or even appendicitis. If the child has a fever, diarrhea, vomiting, lethargy, loss of appetite, or takes to their bed, an infection should be considered and a physician consulted.

Neurological disorder. Seizures and motor and vocal tics as well as Tourette's syndrome occur more commonly in autistic children than nonautistic children. Convulsions and staring episodes may be the result of a seizure disorder. Unusual facial movements, hand mannerisms, or feet shuffling may be the manifestation of an uncontrollable tic. These are usually worsened in stressful situations. Finally, unusual vocalizations, barking, or repeated words may be a sign of an undiagnosed Tourette's syndrome.

Medication side effects. The side effects of many medications can cause behavioral changes in both typical and autistic children.

- Cold medicines containing pseudoephedrine can cause hyperactivity and anxiety.
- Antibiotics such as tetracycline can cause abdominal pain and diarrhea.
- Antidepressants can cause increased anxiety, increased appetite, and disinhibition. (*Disinhibition* is an unusual loss of self-restraint, fear, or inhibition.)

Pain. An autistic child's behavior can be affected by pain. Therefore, common painful situations should be considered when there is a change in behavior. Common painful situations that should be considered include bumps and bruises, bone fractures, impacted wisdom teeth, sinus infections, perianal abscess, ingrown toenails, hemorrhoids, and menstrual pain.

Fear. Autistic children may have an inappropriate fear of people, objects, or events. They may fear water because of the tactile stimulus; they may fear the school bus because of the noise or the smell of the exhaust; they may fear a teacher because of her height or tone of voice. Although these are inappropriate fears, they, nonetheless, need to be identified and corrected, if possible. Autistic children may have appropriate fears that are unappreciated by parents and teachers. They may fear aggressive children in their class, physically or verbally abusive bus drivers, and teacher's aides or cleaning people. Episodes of physical and sexual abuse of disabled children, while unusual, are not unheard of. Unexplained bruises and cuts should be investigated. Physical signs of sexual assault should be investigated thoroughly, even if an alternate excuse is given. Law enforcement agencies should be involved if the parent is suspicious of this type of activity.

Discomfort. Many unusual behaviors of autistic children can have a simple explanation and be resolved easily. Tight or itchy clothing can cause a child to writhe in discomfort or take off their clothes. A song, musical note, or discordant noise can cause the child to hold their ears or have a tantrum whenever entering a room with those sounds. Certain smells, especially strong smells like detergents, alcohol, or gasoline, can cause the child to run away, refuse to eat food, or even vomit.

Every effort should be made in these cases to identify and treat the underlying condition medically before treating the behaviors unnecessarily with sedatives or tranquilizers.

Tight or itchy clothing can cause a child to writhe in discomfort or take off their clothes.

Living with Autism

86. How can I help my other children form a relationship with their autistic sibling?

While relationships between an autistic sibling and a typically developed sibling are more difficult to establish, they can be every bit as loving and satisfying as those between two typical siblings.

Children without a full appreciation of the sensitivities and limitations of an autistic sibling find it difficult to engage that sibling in conversation or play. The effects of being frightened, ignored, or rebuffed by the autistic sibling can impede a good relationship.

It is therefore not surprising that young children unfamiliar with how to speak or play with their autistic sibling may become discouraged by the reactions they encounter and seek their playmates elsewhere.

Parents can encourage a good relationship between the siblings by teaching their typical children about autism and a few simple skills. Indeed, research has shown that not only can siblings learn these basic skills to engage their brother or sister with autism, but can improve their relationship and enjoy it.

To improve the relationship between the siblings, the typical siblings need to learn how autistic children are different from them. Their brother or sister may not enjoy being hugged or touched in a certain way. Loud voices or noises from toys or games may be painful or frightening. Overly complex games or games that depend too much on verbal communication may be inappropriate for the autistic sibling—although this is not the case for all autistic children. This is a trial-and-error process for the parents and the siblings. The learning process can take time and should be approached incrementally. Too much too soon may wear out the children and exhaust the patience of siblings and parents alike. When the typical child gains insight into the autistic sibling's sensitivities and interest levels, the basis for better communication and play is established.

Some skills that the typical sibling can develop to better communicate with their autistic sibling are:

Getting their attention: Autistic children may appear not to hear well because the focus of their interest is elsewhere. Before trying to engage the autistic sibling in play, the typical sibling should get their attention. This can include facing the child and getting them to make eye contact and respond in some way.

Simplifying tasks: When attempting to teach their autistic sibling a new game or athletic skill, it is helpful to break that skill down into a series of simple steps. Each step should be explained clearly and demonstrated if possible.

Giving instructions: Any instructions given should be modulated to the autistic child's ability to comprehend. Short and simple instructions are best. If possible, demonstrating what you want may be helpful. Again, the typical child should be encouraged to be patient.

Praising good performance: When the autistic child does cooperate or performs a skill well, praise is in order. This can take the form of verbal praise, hanging up a drawing on the refrigerator, or providing a treat of some kind. Positive reinforcement is a great motivator for both typical and autistic children.

Parents should remember that during this learning process, the rules of skill development apply to both the typical and autistic child. Parents should be patient with the typical child, encourage their efforts, and praise their success.

87. How can I get my autistic child to exercise?

Exercise is important for the autistic as well as the typical child. Regular aerobic exercise has been demonstrated to decrease anxiety in autistic children, reduces weight, reduces risk for heart disease and diabetes, and engages the child in a constructive use of his time.

Before a parent can encourage their child to exercise, he or she must create a space in the home or yard where the child can safely run and play. Some characteristics that this space should have include:

- This area should be enclosed to prevent wandering, getting lost, or having access to strangers.

Exercise is important for the autistic as well as the typical child.

- This space should be easily accessible to the parent and the child should be visible at all times.
- Recall that the autistic child can be very curious and oblivious to danger. Parents need to be circumspect when choosing or improving a play area. Things that would not present a danger to a typical child might be very dangerous to an autistic child. Therefore, parents should be sure that their child's play area is free of attractive hazards, such as:
  - Dangerous things to fall off of, including natural and manmade structures (tool sheds, rock formations, utility poles, or high-tension wire towers)
  - Dangerous things to climb into or fall into (lakes, rivers, pools, wells, drainage pipes, crawl spaces, electrical closets, sump drains, or natural caves)
  - Dangerous things to play with (sharp objects, cutting tools, power tools, explosives, firearms, cigarette lighters, matches, caustic chemicals, medications, wild or otherwise dangerous animals, or small objects that a child could choke on)

In this area, parents or siblings can devote some time of every day to playing games that require low organization and little equipment, such as "tag" or "hide and seek." Eventually games that involve throwing or catching balls can be introduced and as your child's skills grow, more advanced and physically demanding games can be taught.

If the parents enjoy running, swimming, or cycling, the child should be encouraged to participate. These activities can be enjoyed by the whole family, allowing parents and siblings an opportunity to exercise while supervising the exercise of their autistic child.

In some areas, groups of parents and other volunteers form athletic leagues and sports programs for children with disabilities. These can be great opportunities to teach your child athletic skills and get exercise.

88. I spent time and money childproofing my home when my son was an infant. Do I have to change anything now that he has been diagnosed as autistic?

Childproofing your home is not a novel idea or difficult to accomplish for parents with only typical children. With typical children, a gate at a stairway, a lock on cabinet door, or a plastic cover for an electrical outlet will usually suffice. When the child is a few years older, these precautions and devices can be removed without adverse risk to the child.

For parents of autistic children, "childproofing" your home is much more complex and lasts much longer. The characteristics of autistic children make them high risks for injury in the home. As a group, they can be hyperactive and enjoy climbing, throwing, breaking, jumping, peeling, cutting, pulling down, throwing utensils, plates and cups, sweeping items off surfaces, dumping drawers and bins, and climbing out of or breaking windows. They can be very curious and indifferent to obvious dangers from flames, hot liquids, heights, sharp objects, cutting tools, and the like. Finally, because these behaviors can extend for many years beyond what you could expect from a typical child, autistic children are taller, stronger, and smarter than the toddlers many safety devices are designed to protect. They can force open doors, break windows, reach sliding bolts, open simple locking devices, and put keys in locks that are more complex. Autistic children tend to be very curious and very persistent. Typical children tend to outgrow destructive or dangerous behaviors, whereas autistic children tend to continue to manifest unsafe behavior as they continue to grow. You should never underestimate the creativity and persistence of an autistic child when it comes to defeating safety devices.

Therefore, more attention needs to be paid to safety around the house. Safety does not only lay in changing the environment, but also in changing the knowledge and behaviors of the autistic child, the parents, siblings, and other household members. Everyone should be interested in the safety of your child. Leaving doors or gates open, cigarette lighters around, or firearms unsecured are common ways for other household members to affect the child's safety.

89. Is my home unsafe for my autistic child?

Perform a survey of your house or apartment as well as any yard or play area that your child will spend time in. As you enter each space, review the following list and note what risks to your child the room contains and make a note of each safety risk. Parents should examine each room for the potential of:

Fall injuries: Are there unguarded stairways; access to unlocked or opened windows; stairwells, window wells, and tall furniture that can be climbed on; and access to washing machines or dryers, crawl spaces, sump drains, or wells?

Burn injuries/fires: Could your child get access to matches, lighters, lit candles, open pilot lights for stoves, boilers and burners, stove tops, and burning cigarettes, cigars, or pipes? Can your child open a hot water faucet or touch hot water from boilers, radiators, or heating pipes? Can they reach toasters, teapots, or coffee urns? Are there caustic chemicals, pipe cleaners, solvents, or acids accessible?

Cut injuries: Does the space contain knives, razors, scissors, broken glass or ceramics, saws, garden clippers, weed cutters, lawn mowers, and other power tools?

Suffocation/strangulation/drowning: Can your child grab small swallowable objects, plastic bags, and plastic sheets? Could they get their head or neck caught in hanging ropes, electrical wires, nets, or bars? Do they have access to pools, ponds, lakes, wells, or any other open water?

Electrical injuries: Are there exposed electrical wires; uncovered electrical outlets; electrical appliances that are too near tubs, sinks, or other bodies of water that the child could throw them into?

Toxic ingestions: Are there accessible cleaning fluids, drain cleaners, acids, lye, paint remover, gasoline, kerosene, pesticides, medications, vitamins, minerals, hobby supplies, paint chips, and so forth?

Firearms injury: Are there firearms that are accessible? Even if they appear out of reach or out of sight, they may be found by a curious child.

Elopement: Are there unlocked doors or windows that the child can use to leave the home? If your child left this space, would you notice? Are alarms available for this purpose?

90. How do I make my home safe for my autistic child?

The following suggestions have been found to be helpful in preventing certain types of behaviors and ensuring a safer environment. The suggestions range from using locks for security or limiting access to the individual to labeling every functional item and area in the home with photographs or symbols to assist in communication.

After you have identified all the risks in the home, separate each room into one of three categories:

1. Safe
2. Needs modification
3. No access allowed

Safe rooms are those rooms where the child can spend time with little risk to their safety. Rooms that require modification are rooms where furniture may need to be removed or replaced, electrical outlets covered, or locks put on doors and cabinets. Rooms labeled "no access allowed" are those rooms that contain things that can harm the child, but cannot be modified easily. For example, young autistic children have been known to be injured when climbing into washing machines or dryers. If you have a laundry room, it may be easier to put a lock on the door than to design a way to block access to the washer and dryer. The same could be said for basements filled with power tools or painting supplies.

Modify the most important areas first. Not every parent can afford a complete home security makeover. Therefore, parents should identify those areas where the child spends the most time and work to secure them first. For example, the child's bedroom, bathroom, den, kitchen, and backyard are all good places to start because these are the primary areas of interaction for many children with autism.

Autistic kids can be hard on furniture.

Get the right furniture. Autistic kids can be hard on furniture. They enjoy jumping and climbing; leaping from one piece of furniture to the next. Therefore, high dressers may pose a fall injury, glass-topped coffee tables may be shattered, and sharp edges on end tables can cut and bruise active children. Furniture that poses an immediate risk to the child should be removed from the room. When choosing new furniture for a room that your autistic child will spend a lot of time in (such as their bedroom or playroom), look for soft durable chairs (for example, beanbag chairs), desks and tables with rounded edges, low beds, book cases that can be affixed to the walls, and so forth.

Use locks, fences, and gates where appropriate. It is important to place locks on exterior doors that provide entry or departure to and from the home. For individuals who run away or leave the home without supervision, having locks on the doors can prevent them from leaving. Place locks on interior doors and cabinets where the individual should not have free access, such as cabinets that contain medications or cleaning supplies. Foldable gates can be used to deny access to stairwells or other rooms. Keep in mind that although these gates may be appropriate for small toddlers, as your child gets older and stronger, they may not provide an

Living with Autism

effective barrier. Enclosing the front or backyard with a fence can provide a safe haven for your child to play. If you have a pool, use a cover over the pool and lock it.

Safeguard your windows. If the child likes to climb out of windows, place locks on them. Hardware stores carry special locks for just this purpose. If the child breaks glass or pounds windows, replace the glass panes with Plexiglas to prevent injury. Some parents have had to place wooden boards over windows to prevent injury or elopement.

Use alarms when appropriate. Some autistic kids seem to enjoy escaping from the house unnoticed. They slip out of doors or windows and even open locks as they get older. Putting alarms on doors and windows can alert parents of their child's attempts at escape. This may be safer than putting up too many barriers that may prevent appropriate escape during a house fire. These needn't be expensive, integrated security systems. Local electronic stores sell inexpensive, yet very effective, alarms for individual doors and windows.

Make electrical outlets and appliances safe. Cover or remove electrical outlets and access to electrical appliances. Use plastic knob covers for doors, faucets, ovens, and stove burners. Ensure that all wiring for appliances and electronics is concealed in a way that the child cannot play with the wires or bite or cut them. Heavy items such as televisions, VCRs, or computers should not be stored in high places, so that a child could pull them down on his- or herself.

Lock dangerous items away. Make sure toxic substances are secured in a locked cabinet. These substances include detergents, caustic chemicals, cleaning supplies, pesticides, medications, and small items that a child may mouth or chew. Sharp tools and kitchen implements should locked away (if practical) or placed out of sight and out of easy reach, if they are regularly used.

Rather than have these items all over the house in places that are convenient to the chores they are used for, it may be safer to store them in one place, such as a closet or cabinet that can be securely locked. For items such as kitchen knives or sharp scissors, locks can be placed on individual kitchen cabinets or drawers.

Remember fire safety. Regarding fire safety, it is important to have lighters and matches out of reach or locked up. Place safety covers over gas stoves and oven knobs so the child cannot turn them on. Always supervise the children closely when there is an active fire in the fireplace or when there is a barbeque with open flames. Many community fire departments can provide stickers (often called tot finders) for bedroom windows of children. These are invaluable in the event of a fire, so that firefighters can locate a child's bedroom quickly. Although it may be difficult to teach an individual with autism or PDD about the dangerous nature of fire, it may be possible to teach them about how to behave when it comes to fire safety.

Be careful with firearms in the house. Autistic children will not readily learn gun safety. No guns should be accessible in nightstands, on top of dressers, and the like. All firearms should be locked in a gun safe, unseen and inaccessible to children in the house.

Consider identification options. Autistic children have a tendency to wander, to lag behind groups, to get lost, and sometimes escape from their own home.

If your child has proper identification, it is easier for others to help them return home. This is especially true if your child is unable to communicate effectively. If your child will tolerate wearing a medical ID bracelet or necklace, get one (they can be found at your local drug store or ordered on the Internet). However, many children with autism do not like to wear jewelry, so the next best option is to place iron-on labels into each garment. Some children can be taught to carry an identification card in their wallet, purse, fanny pack, or knapsack. Children can be taught to show their identification cards when asked by adults.

91. How do I change my child's behaviors to reduce risk of accident or injury?

Risks in and out of the home cannot be effectively eliminated; for example, it is impossible to abolish hot cooking pots on the stove, sharp knives in the utensil drawer, or the traffic on busy streets. In these cases, teaching children about the dangers and ways to avoid them is important. Developing social stories about smoke detectors, fire drills, fire alarms, touching fire, talking to strangers, and so forth is the place to begin. (A social story is a short, personalized story that explains the subtle cues in social situations and breaks down a situation or task into easy-to-follow steps.) These stories need not be long or complex, and they should be repeated often, especially in potentially risky situations. For example, when Mom is cooking on the stove, she may tell the story to her child of a boy who burned his hand when he touched the flame or the hot pan. These stories can be embellished with songs, rhymes, or funny faces. However, if repeated often enough, the child will learn to avoid the dangerous situation.

In addition to social stories, the use of visual (photos or pictures) rules can assist the child in understanding what they are not supposed to do and/or what they are expected to do. For example, "no touching the oven burners" with a photograph of the oven burners with a bright red "no" symbol or STOP sign over the photograph may visually depict the rule for the child.

The behavior of the child is not the only behavior that must change.

The behavior of the child is not the only behavior that must change. Parents used to caring for typical children will notice the supervising takes a lot more effort. The parents or guardians of autistic children need to be more vigilant, because autistic children tend to be more persistent in their actions and are not deterred by obvious dangers or chastened by stern lectures.

Children with autism may need extra precautions to stay safe in your home. However, it is important to find a balance between keeping your child secure and making your home a prison. You should keep in mind that locks should not be so secure that they prevent anyone from leaving the house during an emergency such as a fire. Vigilance is an important virtue in the parents of autistic children. Vigilance requires more effort and can induce more stress. Dealing with this stress is discussed in question 96 in this book.

92. Where do autistic people usually live?

In general, autistic people have the same living options as people with other disabilities. Their living arrangements are matched with the individual's needs, capabilities, and the finances of their family. It is important for parents to understand that, unlike educational services, the federal and state governments have no obligation to provide their child with a place to live. Therefore, parents must consider today where they'd like their child to live in the future and begin making plans years before the child will require those arrangements. In the past, autistic children were likely to be placed in an institution. Today, except in rare instances, autistic children live with their parents.

Autistic adults, however, have more options. These options include:

Family home. Parents or interested and involved siblings can provide a home and care for their autistic family member. If the parents have no typical children to care for their child after they die, they can arrange for a caretaker or companion to live with their child in the home.

State-run mental health facility. This is an option for autistic adults with severe intellectual or behavioral impairment who require continual care and supervision. Although the trend in recent decades has been to avoid placing persons with disabilities into long-term care institutions, this alternative is still available when necessary. Unlike many of the institutions years ago, today's facilities view residents as individuals with human needs and offer opportunities for recreation and simple but meaningful work.

Group home. A group home is a single-family residential structure designed or adapted for occupancy by unrelated developmentally disabled persons. The structure provides long-term housing and support services that are residential in nature. The residents typically participate in daily tasks and are often free to come and go on a voluntary basis. A group home might have four permanent residents with two staff members for most of the waking hours and one staff member while the residents sleep. A group home can be owned and funded by the state, a charitable organization, or a family.

Assisted living facility. Assisted living refers to a residential care facility that provides housing, support services, and at times, health care for a group of unrelated developmentally disabled people. Typically, these people are not able to live independently, but do not need the level of care that an institution offers. The assisted living situation can be tailored to the needs of the individuals; for example, two autistic people could share an apartment and be visited daily by a representative of social services. An assisted living facility can be owned and operated by the state, a charitable organization, or a family.

93. What is respite care?

Families caring for a disabled person can be tied down much more than other families. Autistic children are individuals and the amount of supervision autistic children require varies, but in general, there is an extra burden on the parents. This burden can be severe in many cases. Providing care and supervision can possibly require as much effort as would an additional full-time job.

"Respite" or "**respite care**" refers to short-term, temporary care provided for people with disabilities such as autism. This care is given so that their families can take a break from the daily routine of caregiving. Unlike child care, respite services may sometimes involve overnight care or care for an extended period.

Respite care

A short period of rest or relief. Parents of a child with a disability may qualify for respite services when a child is cared for by a third party allowing the parent(s) to take care of other needs away from the child, like the needs of themselves or other children in the family.

215

Respite is often referred to as a gift of time.

One of the important purposes of respite is to give family members time and temporary relief from the stress they may experience while providing extra care for a child with autism. This, in turn, can help prevent increased family stress, support family unity, and avoid child abuse and neglect. Respite care enables families to take vacations or just a few hours of time off. Respite is often referred to as a gift of time.

Respite care services can be provided by other families or friends, charitable groups, or even by government agencies. Most programs are managed by affiliates or chapters of national organizations such as The Arc, Easter Seal Society, and United Cerebral Palsy Associations in cooperation with local hotels. Many other programs are provided by local organizations such as churches, schools, and other nonprofit groups. Sometimes families arrange for care with neighbors or other people they know.

The service may consist of providing an experienced caregiver to look after the child for a few hours; others require that the individual come to a day care center or group home set up to take care of the child for a weekend on occasion.

William's comment:

I wish we used respite. We don't. Not because we don't feel stressed. We do. And not because we don't think that some time alone would help us to relax—we do. Our lives would be a lot easier if we did so. However, we can't bring ourselves to leave Liam alone. It is very difficult to entrust such a sensitive and dependent child to the care of others.

94. How can I tell if my family needs respite care services?

Families with an autistic child can suffer constant stress. Despite this elevated level of stress, many parents may be reluctant to use a respite program, fearing caregivers will not understand or appropriately care for their child. Some families may even question the need for this type of service. Experts recommend that families of children with autism ask themselves these questions to determine if respite services may be helpful or even necessary:

- Is it difficult to find temporary care for my child?
- Does caring for my child interfere with scheduling appointments or completing personal projects?
- Have the demands of caring for my autistic child left me depressed, saddened, or chronically fatigued?
- Is it important that my spouse and I enjoy an evening alone together without the children?
- Does caring and supervision of my child prevent me from getting regular exercise?
- Does caring and supervision of my child prevent me from maintaining relationships with friends and family?
- If I had appropriate care for my autistic child, would I use the time for a special activity with my other children?
- Am I concerned that in the event of a family emergency, there is no one with whom I would feel secure to leave my child?
- Would I feel comfortable having a trained, caring respite provider care for my child?
- Has the family avoided vacations altogether because of the fear and anxiety associated with traveling with the autistic child?

Living with Autism

- Do I avoid going out because I feel I would be imposing on the family and friends who care for my child?

If family members answer "yes" to any of these questions, the family may very well benefit from respite care services.

PART XI

Stress

What are some ways that parents
can reduce their stress?

What can I do about my
children's stress?

More . . .

95. How are parents with autistic children stressed?

To be a parent is to be stressed. Being responsible for children, their behaviors, and their demands for attention, time, and finances can exceed even the most capable parent's abilities. An autistic child adds significantly more stress and unique types of stress to any family.

The sources of stress for parents of autistic children include:

Deficits and behaviors of autism: Research indicates that parents of children with autism experience greater stress than parents of children with mental retardation and Down syndrome. This is the result of the distinct characteristics of autism. Caring for a person who cannot communicate is highly frustrating. Autistic children may not be able to express their basic wants or needs. They cannot tell their parents if they are hungry, thirsty, bored, in pain, or nauseated. When the parents cannot determine their child's needs, they feel frustrated and depressed.

The child's hyperactivity, distractibility, and impulsiveness require a higher level of supervision and physical security and these traits interfere with functioning and learning. Further, this inability to engage in self-directed and appropriate play requires the parents or caregivers to constantly structure the child's time. This structuring imposes similar structure on the parents and siblings.

Family activities such as meals, sports, movies, or quiet relaxation are all colored by the mood and abilities of the autistic child. Such questions as:

- Will he sit through the whole movie?
- Will she eat what everyone else is eating?

- Will he throw food while our guest is at the table?
- Will the noise at the circus be too loud?
- Will we have to leave early?
- Should we even bother going?

All of these deficits and behaviors are physically exhausting for families and emotionally draining.

Finally, spouses often cannot spend time alone due to their extreme parenting demands and the lack of qualified people to watch a child with autism in their absence.

Feelings of grief and loss: Parents of children with autism are grieving the loss of the "typical" child that they expected to have. In addition, parents are grieving the loss of lifestyle that they expected for themselves and family. The feelings of grief that parents experience can be a source of stress due its ongoing nature. The parents of autistic children experience episodes of grief triggered by different life events such as birthdays, holidays, or the graduation or marriage of a peer or sibling.

Finances: An autistic child makes demands on a parent's time, emotions, and finances, much more than a typical child does. Expenses such as evaluations, home programs, adapting the home environment, and various therapies can drain a family's resources. A dual-income family may need to become a single-income family, when one parent gives up his or her job to become the primary caregiver. The specter of future costs of care for an adult child is ever present in the parents' minds and a constant source of worry.

Reactions from society: While parents can be very accepting of an autistic child's behavior at home, this same behavior in public may cause them significant stress. People may stare, make comments, or fail to

Stress

221

understand any mishaps or misbehaviors that may occur. Autistic children, even when behaving well, may be too loud, too active, and too friendly with strangers. When frightened, they may scream; when bored or frustrated, they may throw a tantrum. Memories of these public experiences affect family decision making regarding outings, family events, and vacations.

Feelings of isolation: Families may feel uncomfortable taking their child to the homes of friends or relatives. When there is an obligatory family gathering, such as a holiday, wedding, or funeral, the family's stress level can soar. Ultimately, the family may feel as though they cannot socialize or relate to others. Isolation from their friends, relatives, and community is common for parents of autistic children.

The future: Even well-adapted, well-functioning, and balanced parents become distressed when they think of the future for their child. They may ask: "Who will care for my child when I am gone? Will they care for him as well as I do? Will they understand the subtle signs she shows when she is sick? Will they give him his or her favorite foods? How will I pay for this care? Will his siblings have to care for her?" There are no easy answers for these questions, and the worries attendant to them are always in the back of a parent's mind.

96. What are some ways that parents can reduce their stress?

A normal range of emotions, fears, and concerns go along with raising a child with autism. There is a predictable spectrum of stresses from minor irritations to major life-altering troubles. These current and long-term challenges put you and your other children at an increased risk for depression or stress-related illness. Here are some ways you can approach these issues:

Plan respite care frequently

Stress

- *Learn new ways to relax.* Get involved in a hobby, visit with friends, or practice yoga or meditation.
- *Exercise.* Exercise is an excellent way to take your mind off your troubles, at least for a short time. Research shows that exercise improves the moods and decreases the anxiety level of people who practice it regularly (at least three times per week for at least 30 minutes per session). Exercise also improves your health and is a way to manage your weight.
- *Pay attention to your diet as well as your child's.* Monitor the quality and quantity of the food you and your family eats. Food can easily become a way to satisfy yourself or calm your child, but it comes at the expense of your weight and health. Consult a physician or dietitian if this has become a problem.
- *Utilize respite care.* Respite care provides a break for parents and siblings. Plan respite care frequently; don't use it only when an emergency comes up or when you've become burned out. Regularly planned respite care gives parents and siblings an opportunity to relax and allows the autistic child a chance to interact with someone outside of the family or his or her school.
- *Participate in support groups.* Being active in an autism support group can be very helpful. Support groups for parents and siblings give the family members an opportunity to learn from the experience of others. Parents also benefit from having a sympathetic and nonjudgmental group with which to discuss their challenges and frustrations. The Autism Society of America provides information about support groups in your area. Contact them at www.autism-society.org.

- *Use counseling services if necessary.* Talk with a health professional about whether counseling would help if you or one of your children is having trouble handling the strains related to having a family member with autism.
- *Have a spiritual life.* Individual or family prayer can reduce stress and provide a better outlook on the future.
- *Make to-do lists.* Keeping a daily list of chores can help when planning your day. It encourages focus and adds to a sense of accomplishment.

97. Do some families deal with stress better than others?

When a child is diagnosed with autism, it is not uncommon for parents and other caregivers to become angry, depressed, and frightened. The parents and other family members undergo a grieving process, because their goals, dreams, and ambitions for their child are dashed. They are faced with a new reality; one where the child is emotionally distant, behaviorally volatile, and yet highly dependent for basic care. There are new words for the parents to learn, new schools to attend, and a new home environment to create. It is, in fact, a crisis, and the crisis, puts great stress on the family.

Some families are remarkably adaptable in crises. Yet, other families can find it difficult to cope with the stresses and eventually may succumb to them.

William's comment:

Even in an excellent marriage, one spouse may be better equipped to deal with this crisis than the other. We have found this leads to feelings of stress, anger, and inadequacy.

It can cause tension in an otherwise happy marriage. Increased communication and honesty about feelings can increase understanding between the spouses and lessen the tension. Seeking counseling is not a sign of weakness, but of strength, we have found.

Maladaptive families are unable to achieve a balance between meeting their child's needs and maintaining their own functioning. For example, these families may overindulge their child and foster his or her dependency, while other family members may be ignored or mistreated in an effort to meet the needs of the autistic child. Alternatively, maladaptive families may emotionally abandon their autistic child. They may ignore the existence of the child's disability and delay appropriate treatment and services. In some cases, one family member, such as a mother, accepts all responsibility as the child's caregiver and primary therapist. She cares for all of the child's needs as well as performing the usual household chores and caring for her husband and other children. This mother may find it difficult or impossible to perform all these duties. She may become angry and bitter at the other family members who are not "helping out." The family may feel this is the mother's appropriate role and not understand the amount of work that is required. They may feel like they are intruding or not included in the care of the child. In this situation, the mother and the autistic child become isolated and both suffer in the process. These maladaptive patterns stem from a family's inability to communicate their needs effectively with each other, as well as with care providers or with support networks. Additionally, families like these will fail to seek and accept help. They may feel ashamed by their child's diagnosis or they may feel that personally supervising the autistic child at all times is their primary responsibility. Additionally, these families

Stress

may be inflexible in their social or gender roles. For example, they may feel that only the mother should care for the autistic child and that husbands, siblings, or grandparents should not be involved. Finally, these maladaptive families become very isolated because of the demands of the child. They fail to maintain relationships with friends and family. Because of this, they have no outlets for their anger, frustration, and fear. Their social isolation limits their extended support network, which would be an aid in an emergency. Finally, isolation decreases or eliminates interaction with friends with whom they should be able to relax, unwind, and recharge.

In contrast, the characteristics of successfully adaptive families are:

- **Flexibility** in their roles within the family. While one member may act as the primary caregiver, other members take over some of his or her responsibilities. They offer relief or respite at times and unburden the caregiver or family member, regardless of their traditional social roles.
- They **communicate** with each other and outsiders effectively. These families are able to communicate their need for social support, for occasional respite, or for additional educational or therapeutic services.
- They **seek out and accept help**. These families realize that sometimes the demands of an autistic child are more then they can handle. They are not embarrassed by the illness nor do they think it is some kind of divine retribution. It is important for parents to seek assistance from whatever sources are available. They talk to their health professional and investigate what help is available locally. Family, friends, public agencies, and national or community organizations are all potential resources. Support groups for parents, sib-

lings, and grandparents are available through educational programs, parent resource centers, autism societies, and developmental disabilities offices. In addition, online support is available for family members. A case manager or social worker may help to identify sources of aid as well as help to fill out the paperwork.

Finding other families in the same situation can be helpful.

- They **maintain their relationship** with the community. These families realize that having an autistic child can be isolating. Isolation increases family stress and decreases their life enjoyment as well as the size of their social care network. Therefore, these adaptable families make socializing and downtime an important priority in their scheduling. Finding other families in the same situation can be helpful. It gives a family comfort to know that they are not the only ones experiencing a particularly stressful situation. In addition, families can get useful advice from others struggling with the same challenges.
- They have the **ability to solve problems**. These families use these abilities to identify problems associated with raising an autistic child, to effectively communicate what the problem is, to seek out and find help, and to share responsibilities and not be overwhelmed by them.

This type of family is successful in meeting the needs of their autistic child without a loss of balance and functioning.

98. Do siblings suffer increased stress as a result of having an autistic brother or sister?

Yes, at times, an autistic brother or sister can increase a sibling's stress levels. In fact, research demonstrates that the siblings of children with autism report higher stress levels than siblings of children with other types of disabilities. Common causes of stress for the siblings of autistic children include:

- **Embarrassment.** When in the company of peers, the behaviors of an autistic sibling may cause embarrassment. The sibling may avoid having friends over to the house. They may not discuss their brother or sister's condition or even his or her existence with friends or classmates.

- **Jealousy.** Autistic children can dominate the time and emotional energy of the parents. Some siblings may feel left out, become resentful, or become jealous.

- **Frustration.** Autistic children experience significant problems with socialization and communication. Siblings of these children may experience frustration over not being able to engage or get a response from their brother or sister. Brothers and sisters who would like to play with, comfort, or protect their sibling may become frustrated by their inability to communicate with him.

- **Physical abuse.** Autistic children have limited abilities to show that they are frightened or frustrated. Some may vent this frustration by becoming physically aggressive. Siblings are often a convenient target of this inappropriate expression of frustration. Although this is rarely dangerous for the sibling, it can be extremely upsetting.

- **Self-discipline.** Siblings may become overly sensitive to the burdens placed on the parents by their autistic brother or sister and may try to overcompensate with their own behavior. This attempt at trying to make up for the deficits of their brother or sister may manifest itself by the typical sibling attempting to be especially well behaved or especially successful in athletics or scholastics. This self-imposed discipline may become unrealistic, overly demanding, or abusive.

- **Anxiety about parents**. Children are sensitive to their parents' stress and may fear the consequences of the parents' stress or grief. They may fear for their parents' health, happiness, or the longevity of the marriage. The siblings may ask themselves: "Will my parents fight again? Will they get divorced? Will this cause my father to have a heart attack? What will happen to me?"

- **Fear**. As the siblings grow older, they realize that their autistic sibling requires a lot of care and supervision. Further, they realize that their parents will not be able to care for their autistic sibling forever. They may worry that they may have to care for their brother or sister or may feel guilty because they don't want to become their sibling's primary caregiver. They may fear the future. "Who will care for my brother when my parents are gone? Will I have to care for him? Could I get married if I had to care for my brother? What would my spouse say about it?"

- **Guilt**. Siblings may experience guilt when asking for appropriate things, such as their share of parental attention, time alone, money, or even suggesting a family trip without the autistic sibling.

Not all siblings will experience these issues, but parents and other caregivers should be aware of them and take actions to prevent them when possible.

Like parents, grandparents, uncles, aunts, and cousins can grieve over the loss of the "typical" child they expected. In addition, these family members are concerned about the stress and difficult situations they see the child's parents experiencing.

Many of these family members want to help but don't know how. They are usually inexperienced in caring for autistic children and may be frightened by the prospect. They may not have the energy or the physical strength to manage the child. The usual positive feedbacks that come from sweets, toys, and trips to the zoo appear unappreciated or ignored. This can cause parents to become frustrated when they perceive other family members not understanding their situations or helping out.

99. What can I do about my children's stress?

Some of this stress is an unavoidable aspect of being the sibling of an autistic child and little can be done about it. Careful planning and honest discussion with your children can avoid other stresses. Parents should discuss the common causes of stress and any other issues about their brother or sister that concerns them. They should explain to their children what social and personal situations they can expect and what they should do about it. Parents should encourage open communication about these issues and absolve their children from feelings of guilt and calm their worries when possible. Regularly scheduled respite care for the autistic child allows the families a time to relax and decreases the stress levels of parents and children. When possible, having the children attend formal or informal support groups for the siblings of autistic children gives these siblings an opportunity to see that they are neither alone in their situation nor in their feelings. If these conservative measures fail, having your children discuss their fears and anxieties with a counselor may be helpful.

Although the amount of stress on siblings may be higher than normal, it is not clear that siblings will be adversely affected by it. Existing research studies have shown mixed results relating to the impact upon children of having a sibling with a disability.

In some studies, siblings of children with autism may exhibit more behavior problems than children who don't have a sibling with autism. These behavior problems might include acting out, aggressive behavior, and disobedience. However, research has also found that having a sibling with autism may result in some positive consequences. Some brothers and sisters show a more positive self-concept, higher maturity and empathy levels, and better social skills and adjustment than their peers with typical siblings.

Some brothers and sisters show a more positive self-concept, higher maturity and empathy levels, and better social skills and adjustment than their peers with typical siblings.

Stress

100. Where can I get more information about autism?

There are many resources available to parents of autistic children. These include the support organizations and Web sites found on the following pages. Many more resources are available besides those listed here. Check your local library or Web sites like Amazon.com for books or go to any of the following organizations' Web sites and search for links or resources related to autism.

Organizations

Asperger Syndrome Coalition of the United States (ASC-US)
P.O. Box 2577
Jacksonville, FL 32203-2577
Phone: 904-745-6741
E-mail: aspen@cybermax.net
ASC-US is a national organization providing information and support to individuals, families, and professionals dealing with neurological communication disorders on the autism spectrum including nonverbal learning disabilities, Asperger syndrome, high-functioning autism, semantic-pragmatic disorder, hyperlexia, and PDD-NOS.

Association for Science in Autism Treatment
P.O. Box 7468
Portland, ME 04112-7468
Phone: 207-253-6008
Fax: 207-253-6058
Web site: www.asatonline.org

Autism National Committee (AUTCOM)
35657 Anthony Road
Agua Dulce, CA 91390
E-mail: jeff@jaynolan.org
Web site: www.autcom.org

Autism Network International (ANI)
P.O. Box 35448
Syracuse, NY 13235-5448
E-mail: jisincla@mailbox.syr.edu
Web site: http://ani.autistics.org

Autism Research Institute (ARI)
4182 Adams Avenue
San Diego, CA 92116
Phone: 619-281-7165
Fax: 619-563-6840
Web site: www.autismresearchinstitute.com

Autism Resources Nationwide
Web site: www.autism-info.com

Autism Society of America
7910 Woodmont Avenue, Suite 300
Bethesda, MD 20814-3067
Phone: 301-657-0881; 800-3AUTISM (328-8476)
Fax: 301-657-0869
Web site: www.autism-society.org

Council of Parent Attorneys and Advocates (COPAA)
P.O. Box 81-7327
Hollywood, FL 33081-0327
Phone: 954-966-4489
Web site: www.copaa.net
COPAA is an independent, nonprofit organization of attorneys, advocates, and parents established to improve the quality and quantity of legal assistance for parents of children with disabilities.

Cure Autism Now (CAN) Foundation
5455 Wilshire Blvd., Suite 715
Los Angeles, CA 90036-4234
Phone: 323-549-0500; 888-8AUTISM (828-8476)
Fax: 323-549-0547
E-mail: info@cureautismnow.org
Web sites: www.cureautismnow.org; www.canfoundation.org

DAN! Defeat Autism Now!
Web site: www.autism.com/ari/dan.html

Educational Resources Information Center (ERIC)
1920 Association Drive

Reston, VA 22091-1589
Phone: 703-264-9474; 800-328-0272
http://www.eric.ed.gov/
Information clearinghouse funded by the U.S. Dept. of Education and hosted by the Council for Exceptional Children.

Federation for Children with Special Needs
Web site: www.fcsn.org

Families and Advocates Partnership for Education (FAPE)
Web site: www.fape.org
This is a partnership that aims to improve the educational outcomes for children with disabilities. It links families, advocates, and self-advocates to information about the Individuals with Disabilities Education Act (IDEA). The project is designed to address the information needs of the six million families throughout the country whose children with disabilities receive special education services.

MAAP Services for Autism, Asperger's, and PDD
P.O. Box 524
Crown Point, IN 46308
Phone: 219-662-1311
Fax: 219-662-0638
E-mail: chart@netnitco.net
Web site: www.maapservices.org

MEDLINEplus: Assistive Devices
MEDLINEplus is an online service of the National Library of Medicine. It is designed to link users to information on specific health topics including assistive devices. MEDLINEplus brings together information from many sources and is updated every day. The site includes general information about assistive devices, plus links to information about funding, research, specific conditions, dictionaries, organizations, statistics, and children, teenagers, and seniors. Some information is available in Spanish.
Web site in English: www.nlm.nih.gov/medlineplus/assistivedevices.html
Web site en Español: www.nlm.nih.gov/medlineplus/spanish/assistivedevices.html

National Alliance for Autism Research (NAAR)
99 Wall Street
Research Park
Princeton, NJ 08540
Phone: 609-430-9160; 888-777-NAAR (6227)
California: 310-230-3568
Fax: 609-430-9163
E-mail: naar@naar.org
Web site: www.naar.org

National Autism Hotline
Autism Services Center
605 Ninth Street, Prichard Bldg.
Huntington, WV 25701-0507
Phone: 304-525-8014
Fax: 304-525-8026
Web site: www.autismservicescenter.org

National Center on Birth Defects and Developmental Disabilities (NCBDDD)
Web site: www2.cdc.gov/ncbddd/pubs/KeywordSearch.asp
The NCBDDD staff have written scientific papers on ASD; these papers look at such topics as how common ASD are and vaccines. You can see a list of these papers (starting in 1990) by using the keyword search on the NCBDDD publications Web page. Choose "autism" in the keyword box on the search page. You can choose whether you want the list to be sorted by author or by date. You can also choose to have the list appear with or without graphics. Click on the Submit button. You will see a list of papers that are about ASD. The list will include the complete reference for each paper and a link to an abstract of the paper or to the full text, when available.

National Council on Disability (NCD)
1331 F Street NW, #1050
Washington, D.C. 20004
202-272-2004
This council is an independent federal agency making recommendations to the president and Congress on issues affecting the 54 million Americans with disabilities.

**National Dissemination Center for Children
with Disabilities**
U.S. Dept. of Education, Office of Special Education Programs
P.O. Box 1492
Washington, DC 20013-1492
Phone: 800-695-0285
Fax: 202-884-8441
E-mail: nichcy@aed.org
Web site: www.nichcy.org

**National Information Center on Children and Youth with
Disabilities (NICHCY)**
Phone: 800-695-0285
E-mail: nichcy@aed.org
Web site in English: http://www.nichcy.org/
Web site en Español: www.nichcy.org/pubs/spanish/fs1stxt.htm
NICHCY provides information on disabilities and disability-
related issues for families, teachers, and other professionals.
NICHCY has a fact sheet about autism that includes informa-
tion on topics such as characteristics of children with autism,
the impact of autism on a child's education, and resources.
NICHCY also has a more detailed paper about pervasive devel-
opmental disorders that includes information about all forms of
autism spectrum disorders but focuses mostly on PDD–NOS.
The paper has information on the causes, symptoms, diagnosis,
and treatment of pervasive developmental disorders.

**National Institute of Child Health & Human
Development (NICHD)**
National Institutes of Health, DHHS
31 Center Drive, Room 2A32 MSC 2425
Bethesda, MD 20892-2425
Phone: 301-496-5133
Fax: 301-496-7101
Web site: www.nichd.nih.gov
NICHD has several fact sheets and other publications related to
ASD. Some give basic information about ASD, including
symptoms, causes, and treatment. Others talk about vaccines,
the role of genetics, and programs funded by NICHD. Many
of these materials are available in both English and Spanish.

National Institute on Deafness and Other Communication Disorders Information Clearinghouse
1 Communication Avenue
Bethesda, MD 20892-3456
Phone: 800-241-1044; TTD/TTY: 800-241-1055
E-mail: nidcdinfo@nidcd.nih.gov
Web site: www.nidcd.nih.gov

National Institute of Mental Health (NIMH)
National Institutes of Health, DHHS
6001 Executive Blvd., Room 8184, MSC 9663
Bethesda, MD 20892-9663
Phone: 301-443-4513; 301-443-8431
TTY: 866-615-NIMH (6464)
Fax: 301-443-4279
E-mail: nimhinfo@nih.gov
Web sites: www.nimh.nih.gov; www.nimh.nih.gov/publication/autism.cfm
NIMH has a booklet about autism that includes sections on what autism is, what causes autism and how it is diagnosed, what other disabilities a child with autism may have, what education and treatment programs are available, what research offers, and where to go for information and support.

National Institute of Neurological Disorders and Stroke (NINDS)
Web site in English: www.ninds.nih.gov/health_and_medical/pubs/autism.htm
Web site en Español: www.ninds.nih.gov/health_and_medical/pubs/autismo.htm
NINDS has a fact sheet on autism that includes information on common signs of the condition, diagnosis, causes, treatment, and where to go for more information. The fact sheet includes links to information sheets about pervasive developmental disorders and Asperger disorder.

National Parent to Parent Support and Information System
Web site: www.nppsis.org

S.N.A.P. (Special Needs Advocate for Parents)
Web site: www.snapinfo.org

West Coast Office:
1801 Avenue of the Stars, #401
Century City, CA 90067
Phone: 888-310-9889; 310-201-9614

East Coast Office:
30A Vreeland Road, Suite 130
Florham Park, NJ 07932
Phone: 877-348-6497; 973-236-9887
S.N.A.P. is a nonprofit public benefit corporation that provides information, education, advocacy, and referrals to families with special needs children of all ages and disabilities.

National Center for Law and Learning Disabilities (NCLLD)
P.O. Box 368
Cabin John, MD 20818
Phone: 301-469-8308
Web site: www.his.com/~plath3/nclld.html
NCLLD is a nonprofit organization that provides education, advocacy, and analysis of legal issues, policy recommendations, and resource materials.

**National Association of Protection and Advocacy
Systems (NAPAS)**
900 Second Street, NE, Suite 211
Washington, DC 20002
Phone: 202-408-9514
Web site: www.protectionandadvocacy.com
The association provides literature on legal issues and referrals to federally mandated programs that advocate for the rights of people with disabilities.

National Resources for Children with Disabilities
Web site: www.childrenwithdisabilities.ncjrs.org/national.html
This is a great place to locate resources for advocacy, education, technical assistance, and more.

National Alliance for Autism Research (NAAR)
99 Wall Street, Research Park
Princeton, NJ 08540
Phone: 609-430-9160; 888-777-NAAR (6227)
Fax: 609-430-9163

E-mail: naar@naar.org
Web site: www.naar.org
NAAR is a national nonprofit organization for ASD. The NAAR supports research to find the causes of ASD and to prevent, treat, and ultimately cure them. The Web site provides information and current research about ASD, as well as many links to other organizations.

Siblings for Significant Change
350 Fifth Ave., Room 627
New York, NY 10118
Phone: 212-643-2663; 800-841-8251
Web site: www.archrespite.org/archfs23.htm
This is a national network that works to build mutual support for siblings of handicapped persons. They train siblings to be advocates for themselves and their families and provide networking for support and socializing, quarterly meetings, newsletter, phone network, speakers bureau, audio-visual material, and local chapters.

Office of Disability Employment Policy (ODEP)
Department of Labor
200 Constitution Avenue, NW
Washington, D.C. 20210
Phone: 202-376-6200; 866-487-2365 (Department of Labor)
DOL TTY: 877-889-5627. Spanish operators available.
E-mail: infoODEP@dol.gov
Web site: www.dol.gov/odep
The Office of Disability Employment Policy (formerly the President's Committee on Employment of People with Disabilities) provides information, training, and technical assistance to America's business leaders, organized labor, rehabilitation and other service providers, advocacy organizations, families, and individuals with disabilities. ODEP's mission is to facilitate the communication, coordination, and promotion of public and private efforts to empower Americans with disabilities through employment. ODEP also serves as an advisor to the president of the United States on public policy issues affecting employment of people with disabilities.

Social Security Administration (SSA)

Web site: www.ssa.gov/work; Spanish materials available

The Social Security Administration's Work Site provides clarity on matters affecting the employment of Social Security beneficiaries with disabilities. The site contains the latest news on proposed policy changes, upcoming events, and other initiatives related to the Work Incentives Improvement Act of 1999.

Department of Vocational Rehabilitation

Web site: www.jan.wvu.edu/SBSES/VOCREHAB.htm

Vocational rehabilitation (VR) is a nationwide federal-state program for assisting eligible people with disabilities to define a suitable employment goal and become employed. Each state capital has a central VR agency, and there are local offices in most states. VR provides medical, therapeutic, counseling, education, training, and other services needed to prepare people with disabilities for work. VR is an excellent place for a youth or adult with a disability to begin exploring available training and support service options. For more information, contact your child's special education teacher or guidance counselor.

Vocational rehabilitation (VR)

A federal program that provides transition support for eligible students who receive special education services in high school. Referral to vocational rehabilitation is determined by the IEP team during the student's junior year in high school.

Glossary

Accommodations: Changes in curriculum or instruction that do not substantially modify the requirements of the class or alter the content standards or benchmarks. Accommodations are determined by the individual educational plan (IEP) team and are documented in the student IEP.

Addiction theory of autism: The belief that an overabundance of naturally produced opioid compounds (called endorphins or encephalins) are the cause of autism.

Americans with Disabilities Act (ADA): A federal civil rights law passed in 1990. It prohibits discrimination on the basis of disability in (1) employment; (2) programs, services, and activities of state and local government agencies; and (3) goods, services, facilities, advantages, privileges, and use of places of public accommodation.

Annual goals: A set of general statements that represent expected achievement over a year's time for children with disabilities enrolled in special education programs and services. These are stated in the child's IEP.

Applied behavioral analysis (ABA): A system of early educational intervention first developed by Ivar Lovaas. It uses a series of trials to shape a desired behavior or response. Skills are broken down into their simplest components and then taught to the child through a system of reinforcement. It is designed to promote appropriate language and behaviors and to reduce problematic ones.

Asperger syndrome (AS): A developmental disorder on the autism spectrum defined by impairments in communication and social development and by narrow interests and repetitive behaviors. Unlike typical autism, individuals with Asperger syndrome have no significant delay in language or cognitive development. People with Asperger syndrome have difficulty with social understanding, and their patterns of behavior are often inflexible. Language, and especially abstract language, can be hard for these people.

Attention deficit hyperactivity disorder (ADHD): A disorder of childhood and adolescence characterized by lack of impulse control, inability to concentrate, and hyperactivity. A particular symptom complex with core symptoms including developmentally inappropriate degrees of attention, cognitive disorganization, distractibility, impulsivity, and hyperactivity, all of which vary in different situations and at different times. Also called attention deficit disorder (ADD).

Atypical antipsychotic medications: A group of drugs that are different chemically from the older drugs used to treat serious mental illnesses. They are called atypical because they have different side effects than the conventional antipsychotic agents. The atypical drugs are less likely to cause drug-induced involuntary movements than are the older drugs. They may also be effective for some conditions that are resistant to older drugs. The drugs in this group are clozapine (Clozaril), loxapine (Loxitane), olanzapine

(Zyprexa), quetiapine (Seroquel), and risperidone (Risperdal).

Atypical autism: A general term for conditions that are close to but don't quite fit the set of conditions for autism or other specific conditions. This condition is also referred to as pervasive developmental disorder–not otherwise specified or PDD–NOS.

Audiogram: The graphic record drawn from the results of hearing tests with an audiometer, which charts the threshold of hearing at various frequencies against sound intensity in decibels.

Autism: A developmental disturbance that is characterized by an abnormal or impaired development in social communication and interaction skills and significantly restricted range of activities and interests.

Autistic regression: A loss of previously acquired skills including language, sociability, play, and cognition. This regression occurs in about one third of autistic children. The cause of this regression is unknown.

Autistic savants: Autistic individuals who display incredible aptitude for one or two skills (e.g., amazing musical or art ability).

Autism spectrum disorders: A term that encompasses autism and similar disorders. More specifically, the following five disorders listed in the *DSM–IV*: Autistic disorder, Asperger syndrome, pervasive developmental disorder–not otherwise specified, childhood disintegrative disorder, and Rett syndrome.

Behavioral disorders: Disorders affecting behavior and emotional well-being.

Beriberi: A specific nutritional deficiency syndrome that occurs from a deficiency of thiamine. It results in painful nerve damage in the hands and feet and heart failure.

Causal relationship: A correlation between two variables where a change in the first variable causes a change in the second.

Celiac disease (CD): A disease in which the intestinal lining becomes inflamed after ingestion of foods containing gluten (a protein found in oats, wheat, rye, barley, and triticale). The symptoms in infants and children include diarrhea, slow growth, bloody stools, weight loss, and vomiting. Thought erroneously to be a cause of autism.

Centers for Disease Control and Prevention (CDC): A federal agency in the Department of Health and Human Services; located in Atlanta, Georgia; investigates, diagnoses, and tries to control or prevent diseases (especially new and unusual diseases).

Centers for Medicare and Medicaid Services (CMS): Formerly the Health Care Financing Administration; in the U.S. Department of Health and Human Services; the federal agency charged with overseeing and approving states' implementation and administration of the Medicaid program.

Checklist for Autism in Toddlers (CHAT): A checklist to be used by general practitioners at 18 months to see if a child has autism.

Chelating agent: An organic compound in which atoms form more than one chemical bond with metals in solution.

Chelation: The formation of a complex between a metal ion and two or more polar groupings of a single molecule. For example in heme, the Fe^{2+} ion is chelated by the porphyrin ring. Chelation can be used to remove an ion from participation in biological reactions, as in the chelation of Ca^{2+} of blood by EDTA, which thus acts as an anticoagulant. A chelating agent will bind with metals in order to try to release them from the body.

Child psychiatrist: A physician (medical doctor) specializing in mental, emotional, or behavior disorders in children and adolescents; is qualified to prescribe medications.

Child psychologist: A mental health professional with a doctorate in psychology who administers tests, evaluates, and treats children's emotional disorders; cannot prescribe medication.

Childhood Autism Rating Scale (CARS): An autism screening test developed at Treatment and Education of Autistic and Related Communication-Handicapped CHildren (TEACCH). The child is rated in 15 areas on a scale up to 4 yielding a total up to 60; ranges are considered to be nonautistic, autistic, and severely autistic.

Childhood disintegrative disorder (CDD): A condition occurring in 3- and 4-year-olds characterized by a deterioration of intellectual, social, and language functioning from previously normal functioning. Children with this condition, which is sometimes misdiagnosed as autism, develop normally for a prolonged period of time, but then experience loss of social skills, bowel and bladder control, play behaviors, receptive and expressive language, motor skills, and nonverbal communication skills.

Chromosomes: Structures in the cell nucleus that bear an individual's genetic information.

Cognitive: A term that describes mental processes by which the sensory input is transformed, stored, and retrieved.

Cognitive development: The development of the functions of the brain including perception, memory, imagination, and use of language.

Comprehensive evaluation: A series of tests and observations, formal and informal, conducted for the purpose of determining eligibility for special education and related services and for determining the current level of educational performance.

Congenital: Any trait or condition that exists from birth.

Convulsions: Involuntary spasms especially those affecting the full body.

Coprolalia: The involuntary uttering of vulgar or obscene words.

Developmental delays: A term used to describe the development of children who have not reached various milestones in the time frame that is typical for children of his or her chronological age; may occur in one or more areas of functioning.

Developmental disability (DD): A disability of a person manifested before the age of 22 and expected to continue indefinitely. Attributable to mental retardation, cerebral palsy, epilepsy, autism, brain injury, or another neurological condition closely related to mental retardation or requiring treatment similar to that required for mental retardation; results in substantial functional limitations in three or more major areas of life activity.

Developmental regression: A form of autism in which infants, after apparently normal development, start to lose language and other skills. This condition is fairly rare and has not been well described nor does it have scientifically established standards for diagnosis.

Diagnosis: Identification of a disease, disorder, or syndrome through a method of consistent analysis.

Diagnostic and Statistical Manual (DSM-IV): The official system for classification of psychological and psychiatric disorders prepared and published by the American Psychiatric Association.

Disability: A personal limitation or challenge that represents a substantial disadvantage when attempting to function in society; should be considered within the context of the environment, personal factors, and the need for individualized supports.

Discrete trial: A short, instructional exercise that has three distinct parts: e.g., a direction, a behavior, a consequence.

Down syndrome: A genetic condition in which an individual has 47 chromosomes instead of 46; typically characterized by physical anomalies and developmental delays; it is the most frequently occurring chromosomal disorder.

Early intervention: Specific services that are provided to infants and toddlers who show signs of, or are at risk of, having a developmental delay. These services are often tailored to the specific needs of each child with the goal of further-ing development. Early intervention services are often provided at no cost to children who qualify and their families.

Echolalia: Repetitive words or phrases that autistics may say sometimes hours after the event. Delayed echolalia can occur days or weeks after hearing the word or phrase. Sometimes this will just be an echoed word. Some autistics will mimic whole sentences or even conversations; they may even use convincing accents and the voices of other people.

Electroencephalogram (EEG): A test that uses electrodes placed on the scalp to record electrical brain activity. It is often used to diagnose seizure disorders or to look for abnormal brain wave patterns.

Emotional reciprocity: An impaired or deviant response to other people's emotions; lack of modulation of behavior according to social context; and/or a weak integration of social, emotional, and communicative behaviors.

Endorphins: Naturally produced opiate-like substances implicated in the regulation of pain perception, social and emotional behaviors, and motor activity. Once thought to be a cause of autism.

Epidemiology: The part of medical science that deals with the incidence, distribution, and control of disease in a population.

Epilepsy: A neurological disorder that can lead to convulsions, partial and full loss of consciousness, and absences. It occurs more frequently in autistic people and their families than in the general population.

Etiology: The study of the causes or origins of a disease.

Extended school year services: Special education and related services provided to a qualified student with disabilities beyond the normal school year, in accordance with the student's IEP, and at no cost to the parent of the child. The need for extended services is determined by the student's IEP team.

Facilitated communication: A discredited therapeutic method that employs a person (the facilitator) and an assistive communication device to help autistic children to communicate and eventually overcome autistic behaviors. This theory lacks scientific support. Also known as facilitated communication training.

Fragile X syndrome: A genetic disorder that shares many of the characteristics of autism. Individuals can be tested for Fragile X by having a chromosome test performed.

Gene: Originally defined as the physical unit of heredity, it is probably best defined as the unit of inheritance that occupies a specific locus on a chromosome, the existence of which can be confirmed by the occurrence of different allelic forms. Genes are formed from DNA, are carried on the chromosomes, and are responsible for the inherited characteristics that distinguish one individual from another. Each human individual has an estimated 100,000 separate genes.

Gilliam Autism Rating Scale (GARS): This is a screening checklist designed to be used by parents, teachers, and professionals to help to identify autistic children.

Gluten-free/casein-free diet: A diet believed by some to help improve the symptoms of autism. It involves elimination of gluten (a protein found in wheat and other grains) and casein (a protein found in milk) from the diet. It is believed, although not proven, that the undigested portion of these proteins acts like a chemical in the brain, producing symptoms in children with autism. No scientific evidence supports this theory.

Goiter: A chronic enlargement of the thyroid gland, occurring in areas where food is produced in soil that is low in iodine. Sometimes called struma.

Gross motor: Movement that involves balance, coordination, and large muscle activity.

Guardian: An individual who has been entrusted by the law for the care of another person, for his or her estate (finances), or for both.

Haloperidol: A medication that has been found to decrease symptoms of agitation, hyperactivity, aggression, stereotyped behavior, and affective lability.

High-functioning autism (HFA): Individuals with autism who are not cognitively impaired. Sometimes used as a synonym of Asperger syndrome.

Hypersensitive: Excessive sensitivity to sensations or stimuli.

Hypotonia: Decreased muscle tone.

Individualized education plan (IEP): A team-developed, written program that identifies therapeutic and educational goals and objectives needed to appropriately address the educational needs of a school-aged student with a disability; a plan that identifies the student's specific learning expectations and outlines how the school will address these expectations through appropriate special education programs and services. It also identifies the methods by which the student's progress will be reviewed. For students 14 years or older, it must also contain a plan for the transition to postsecondary education, the workplace, or to help the student live as independently as possible in the community.

Individuals with Disabilities Education Act (IDEA): Federal law that grants entitlement for special education services to children with disabilities.

Interventions: Types of traditional or nontraditional treatments that

may be effective in reducing autistic behaviors.

Landau-Kleffner syndrome: A syndrome characterized by a progressive loss of the ability to understand language and use speech, following a period of normal speech development. It is accompanied by seizure activity and is typically diagnosed through a sleep EEG. Also known as acquired aphasia with convulsive disorder.

Least restrictive environment (LRE): A federal mandate that, to the maximum extent appropriate, children with disabilities be educated with children who are not disabled. This means that the separation of children with disabilities from regular education buildings, programs, and students occurs only as much as necessary to meet the unique needs of special education students.

Mainstreaming: The concept that students with disabilities should be integrated with their nondisabled peers to the maximum extent possible, when appropriate to the needs of the child with a disability. Mainstreaming is one point on a continuum of educational options. The term is sometimes used synonymously with inclusion.

Measles, mumps, and rubella (MMR) vaccine: A vaccine against measles, mumps, and rubella given to children at 18 months and again at around 4 years. Some parents believe it to be directly responsible for autism developing in their child.

Medicaid: Title XIX of the federal Social Security Act and 42 CFR 430 to 456; pays for medical care for low-income persons; is a state-administered program.

Medicare: Title XVIII of the federal Social Security Act and 42 CFR 405 to 424; insurance-like payments for medical care of persons aged 65 and over; administered by federal Social Security Administration.

Mentally retarded (MR): A person with a low cognitive ability or low IQ. Also known as mental retardation.

MRI (magnetic resonance imaging): A diagnostic tool that uses radiofrequency waves and a strong magnetic field rather than X-rays to provide remarkably clear and detailed pictures of internal organs and tissues.

Multidisciplinary evaluation team (MET): A minimum of two persons who are responsible for conducting a comprehensive evaluation of students suspected of being handicapped or children with disabilities being reevaluated.

Multidisciplinary team: A team whose members come from multiple disciplines; they interact and rely on the others for information and suggestions.

Naltrexone: This drug blocks brain cell receptors for opioids. They can also block endorphins, the natural opium-like substances produced by the body that may be abnormally high in autism.

National Institutes of Health (NIH): Located in Bethesda, Maryland, it is the largest governmental medical research center. It is part of the U.S. Department of Health and Human Services. It is composed of 27 separate institutes and is charged with the mission to improve the health of the people of the United States.

Neuroleptic: A class of drug that includes Haldol and Risperdal. Also called antipsychotic medication.

Neurologists: Doctors specializing in medical problems associated with the nervous system.

Nonverbal: There are two types of interpersonal communication: verbal and nonverbal. Nonverbal communication includes information that is transmitted without words, through body language, gestures, facial expressions, or the use of symbols.

Obsessive-compulsive disorder (OCD): Having a tendency to perform certain repetitive acts or ritualistic behavior in an attempt to relieve anxiety.

Occupational therapists: Individuals who specialize in the analysis of purposeful activity and tasks to minimize the impact of disability on independence in daily living. The therapist then helps the family to better cope with the disorder by adapting the environment and teaching subskills of the missing developmental components.

Occupational therapy (OT): A type of treatment that assists in the individual's development of fine motor skills that aid in daily living. It also can focus on sensory issues, coordination of movement and balance, and on self-help skills such as dressing, eating with a fork and spoon, grooming, and the like. It can also address issues pertaining to visual perception and hand-eye coordination.

Pediatrician: A medical doctor who specializes in the treatment and care of infants, children, and adolescents.

Pellagra: A specific nutritional deficiency syndrome that occurs from a deficiency of niacin. It results in gastrointestinal disturbances, skin rashes, and mental disorders. Sometimes called St. Ignatius Itch or alpine scurvy.

Perseveration: This refers to a persistent and often purposeless repetition of speech or movement.

Pervasive developmental disorders (PDD): These are a group of neurologic disorders of unknown cause that are marked by impairment in developmental areas such as social interaction and communication or stereotyped behavior, interests, and activities. The disorders include autistic disorder, Rett syndrome, childhood disintegrative disorder, Asperger syndrome, and pervasive developmental disturbances–not otherwise specified.

Pervasive developmental disorder–not otherwise specified (PDD–NOS): One of the five diagnoses in the autistic spectrum of diseases. The diagnosis of PDD–NOS is used when there is severe impairment in social interaction and verbal and nonverbal communication skills or when stereotyped behavior, interests, and activities are present, but symptoms do not meet the criteria for other autistic disorders.

Physical therapist (PT): A licensed health professional who applies principles, methods, and procedures for analyzing motor or sensorimotor functions to determine the educational significance of the identified areas including areas such as mobility and positioning in order to provide planning, coordination, and the implementation of strategies for eligible individuals.

Pica: A perverted or inappropriate appetite for substances not fit as food. These nonfood items include substances that have no nutritional value, such as clay, dried paint chips, starch, or ice.

Picture Exchange Communication System (PECS): A system created to aid the communication of nonverbal autistic patients. PECS employs a simple picture card system used to encourage autistic people to communicate their needs.

Prevalence: The proportion of people with a particular condition or disease within a given population at a given time.

Prognosis: The possible outcomes of a condition or a disease and the likelihood that each one will occur.

Psychologist: A specialist in one or more areas of psychology; a field of science that studies the mind and behaviors. Areas of specialty can include psychological testing and practitioners of therapy or counseling.

Psychosis: A mental and behavioral disorder causing gross distortion or disorganization of a person's mental capacity, affective response, and capacity to recognize reality.

Refrigerator mother: A phrase in Freudian psychological theory that was used to describe mothers who acted coldly toward their children. This behavior was once erroneously thought to be the cause of (infantile) autism.

Respite care: A short period of rest or relief. Parents of a child with a disability may qualify for respite services when a child is cared for by a third party allowing the parent(s) to take care of other needs away from the child, like the needs of themselves or other children in the family.

Risperdal: Generic name: risperidone. Risperdal, an atypical antipsychotic medication, is designed to block the effects of serotonin and dopa-mine, two neurotransmitter chemicals, in the brain. Conventional antipsychotics seem to affect only dopamine.

Rubella: German measles.

Schizoid personality traits: The traits associated with schizoid personality disorder; these traits include social withdrawal, emotional coldness, aloofness or restriction, and indifference to others.

Schizophrenia: A psychotic disorder characterized by loss of contact with the environment, by noticeable deterioration in the level of functioning in everyday life, and by disintegration of personality expressed as disorder of feeling, thought (as in hallucinations and delusions), and conduct.

Scurvy: A specific nutritional deficiency syndrome characterized by weakness, anemia, swelling of the hands and feet, and ulceration of the gums and loss of the teeth. It is caused by a diet lacking in vitamin C. Also called scorbutus and sea scurvy.

Secretin: A polypeptide neurotransmitter (chemical messenger); one of the hormones that controls digestion, increasing the volume and bicarbonate content of secreted pancreatic juices.

Seizure disorder: Includes any condition of the brain in which there are repeated seizures or convulsions.

Selective serotonin reuptake inhibitor (SSRI): A class of drugs used as antidepressants. Functionally, they increase the levels of serotonin in the body. These drugs can be dangerous if mixed with other drugs such as other antidepressants, illicit drugs, some antihistamines, antibiotics, and calcium-channel blockers. Some examples of SSRIs are Prozac, Zoloft, and Paxil.

Self-injurious behavior (SIB): Self-inflicted bodily harm; harm done to the self by an individual. Individuals with an autistic spectrum disorder are often prone to self-injurious behavior.

Self-stimulatory behaviors (stims): This is the name given to the purposeless repetitive actions that some autistic people feel compelled to do. Examples are hand flapping, spinning, toe walking, and so forth.

Sensory integration (SI): This is a term applied to the way the brain processes sensory stimulation or sensation from the body and then translates that information into specific, planned, coordinated motor activity. Information is received from both internal and external environments through the five senses of vision, touch, taste, hearing, and smell. Our senses are integrated when the nervous system directs this information to the appropriate parts of the brain that enables an individual to attain skills.

Serotonin: A neurotransmitter implicated in the behavioral-physiological processes of sleep, pain and sensory perception, motor function, appetite, learning, and memory.

Social communication: Refers to language that is used in social situations. During the school years, this refers to a child's ability to use language to interact with others in a host of situations, from entering peer groups to resolving conflicts.

Social skills: Defined as the cognitive and overt behaviors a person uses in interpersonal interactions and can range from simple nonverbal behaviors such as eye contact and head nods to the complex verbal behavior of offering a compromise that will meet everyone's needs.

Special education: Specially designed instruction that meets the unique educational needs of the student with disabilities.

Special needs: The unique, out-of-the-ordinary concerns created by a person's medical, physical, or mental, condition. Additional services are usually needed to help a person in one or more of the following areas: thinking, communication, movement, getting along with others, and taking care of his or herself.

Stereotyped behaviors: A common finding with autistic patients. These are repetitive, apparently nonfunctional behaviors, such as rocking and hand flapping;

behaviors in an individual that are repeated many times.

Supplemental Security Income (SSI): A federal assistance program administered by the Social Security Administration for aged, blind, and disabled persons under Title XVI of the Social Security Act to guarantee a certain level of income. SSI recipients have contributed nothing or not enough to the Social Security System to be able to receive benefits on their own earnings record.

Tactile: Related to the sense of touch.

Thimerosal: A compound containing around 50 percent ethylmercury by volume. It is used in vaccines to prevent bacterial and fungal growth.

Tourette's syndrome: An inherited, neurological disorder characterized by repeated and involuntary body movements (tics) and uncontrollable vocal sounds. In a minority of cases, the vocalizations can include socially inappropriate words and phrases; this is called coprolalia. These outbursts are neither intentional nor purposeful. Involuntary symptoms can include eye blinking, repeated throat clearing or sniffing, arm thrusting, kicking movements, shoulder shrugging, or jumping. The disturbance causes marked distress or significant impairment in social, occupational, or other important areas of functioning.

Transition services: A coordinated set of activities that promote movement from school to postschool education, vocational training, integrated employment (including supported employment), continuing and adult education, adult services, independent living, or community participation. Transition goals are determined by the IEP team beginning at age 14 and are based on student and family vision, preferences, and interests.

Treatment and Education of Autistic and Related Communication-Handicapped CHildren (TEACCH): A structured educational program that targets both the strengths and weaknesses that are often seen in children with autism. It is a project of the University of North Carolina.

Tuberous sclerosis: A disorder of the skin and nervous system characterized by mental retardation, seizures, skin lesions, and intracranial lesions. It is caused by a dominant gene and occurs in 1 in 7,000 births.

Tympanogram: The graphic record of a test of the flexibility of the eardrum. It is part of a standard hearing evaluation.

Vocational Rehabilitation (VR): A program that provides transition supports for eligible students who receive special education services in high school. Referral to vocational rehabilitation is determined by the IEP team during the student's junior year in high school.

Index

Index